APPROACHES TO TEACHING IN THE HEALTH SCIENCES

HAROLD J. KNOPKE, PH.D.

NANCY L. DIEKELMANN, R.N., M.S.

ADDISON-WESLEY
PUBLISHING COMPANY
Reading, Massachusetts • Menlo Park, California
London • Amsterdam • Don Mills, Ontario • Sydney

ISBN 0-201-01656-7
ABCDEFGHIJ-MA-798

TO SHEILA AND JOHN

INTRODUCTION
KNOWING WHERE
TO BEGIN

After accepting an appointment, new faculty members are sometimes given three months, a month, or perhaps only a week to prepare for the role of teacher. Whether the role is a new or familiar one, new faculty members have to organize instructional activities, meet and discuss with students, assign grades, and work with other people. Many questions arise, such as how to organize and teach a new course or content unit or how to deal with initial feelings of anxiety about teaching. What if a student asks a question the *first* day and the teacher cannot answer it? What if half of the students stop attending class once the course is in progress (or *want* to stop attending)? What if . . . ?

This book is offered as a guide to teachers in the health sciences. It was written particularly for the new teacher, although it should prove just as useful for experienced teachers. Admittedly, no one book can prepare someone adequately for the teaching experience; however, by providing some basic answers to common questions, this book may help teachers avoid many of the most common and unnecessary mistakes and, at the same time, make the experience more productive, satisfying, and enjoyable.

Teachers will find the book most helpful if they first establish a list of personal educational priorities. These will vary, of course, according to the individual teacher and setting. A new teacher teaching a course in the health sciences, for example, may feel unskilled in this new role, although quite comfortable with the content area to be taught. Another teacher may have completed a few years of teaching and is now able to identify areas within a course or instructional approach that need strengthening. An experienced teacher, on the other hand, might be interested in new techniques to revise and further develop a course or unit of study. The setting may vary as well, from a diploma nursing program to a physical therapy curriculum to a medical school basic science sequence. Whatever their needs, all types of teachers should find this book useful in some way, for it presents some approaches to teaching that represent the practical application of theory and the results of research based on theory. The educational principles and practices discussed are applicable across situations and experience levels.

Chapter 1 is directed specifically toward the new teacher in the health sciences. It discusses initial approaches to new teaching responsibilities, as well as some of the reactions and feelings people commonly experience in their new role as teacher. Chapter 2 presents an overview of the basic approach to teaching this book advocates and summarizes the activities involved in planning, developing, managing, and evaluating the teaching-learning process. The chapters comprising Unit 1 discuss the elements of the planning process that form the foundation for teaching. Unit 2 deals with developmental activities, from producing media resources to constructing learning packages. Unit 3 focuses on the activities and skills that characterize a teacher's contributions to the teaching-learning process. Chapters in this unit examine a range of topics, from lecturing to conducting clinical experiences to developing group skills. Unit 4 concentrates on evaluation, and Unit 5 discusses the role of teachers and how they might develop their relationships with students, colleagues, and themselves.

Teachers of any level of experience should view these chapters as guides for beginning further investigation into specific areas. For those interested in more in-depth information, annotated bibliographies conclude each unit; the listed entries generally represent cogent, easily accessible references that can be used to develop breadth and depth in specific areas. Some material that is readily available elsewhere has purposely not been included in this text. Later chapters suggest how available resources can be incorporated into the teaching development process. Teachers therefore may find it useful to begin with the reference and resource materials listed; as their talents as teachers become increasingly refined, they may then pursue the educational literature in more detail.

Teaching is a growth process and, as such, is highly individualistic. There is no one "right" way of teaching. The approaches, techniques, and suggestions presented here have proved useful for others; individual teachers must decide what is best for themselves and their own teaching situations.

CONTENTS

1 THE NEW TEACHER IN THE HEALTH SCIENCES   1
2 APPROACHING THE RESPONSIBILITIES OF TEACHING   8

UNIT 1
THE PLANNING PROCESS

3 PLANNING TO TEACH   27
4 ASSESSING STUDENT CHARACTERISTICS   43

UNIT 2
THE DEVELOPMENT PROCESS

5 INSTRUCTIONAL MEDIA   57
6 SIMULATION GAMES   78
7 LEARNING PACKAGES   91

UNIT 3
THE MANAGEMENT PROCESS

8 TRADITIONAL TEACHING STRATEGIES   106
9 PERSONALIZED INSTRUCTION   125
10 GROUP SKILLS   132

UNIT 4
THE EVALUATION PROCESS

11 PLANNING FOR EVALUATION   149
12 ASSESSING STUDENT LEARNING   168
13 ASSESSING THE TEACHING-LEARNING PROCESS   186
14 REQUIREMENTS FOR USING THE RESULTS OF EVALUATION   201

UNIT 5
PERSONAL MANAGEMENT

15   TEACHER-STUDENT RELATIONSHIPS   215
16   TEACHER-PEER RELATIONSHIPS   223
17   TEACHER-SELF RELATIONSHIPS   232

INDEX   241

1

THE NEW TEACHER IN THE HEALTH SCIENCES

It is often difficult to know exactly where to begin, where to concentrate efforts, or where to find help when preparing to teach in the health sciences for the first time. New teachers should realize that such difficulties are encountered to varying degrees by beginning and by experienced teachers alike, regardless of academic discipline or professional experience. They should also realize that such difficulties can be met and overcome in several ways, whether through discussions with peers, established teachers, department heads or supervisors; consultation of available educational resources; or participation in their institution's educational development activities.

This book is intended to serve as one educational resource available to teachers in the health sciences. One of its basic tenets is that adult students should not be "spoon-fed," particularly in the health sciences, but should be responsible for their own learning. Thus, its fundamental purpose is to discuss a variety of approaches to teaching that encourage students to fulfill this responsibility.

To accomplish this objective, many of the suggestions and techniques offered deviate from the traditional lecture-demonstration methods most teachers experienced when they were students. For this reason, much that is presented may not be immediately accepted by a teacher's colleagues and students and may even lead to some initial resistance, hostility, or frustration. These reactions subside when the success of well-prepared teaching efforts becomes apparent, for students and colleagues then recognize that what is being done not only makes good educational sense, but good professional sense as well.

PRELIMINARY CONSIDERATIONS

The discussions presented in subsequent chapters are structured according to a four-stage framework for approaching the teaching-learning transaction with students. The general approaches and the specific techniques and activities incorporated in the framework represent various aspects of teaching programs conducted by effective teachers.

New teachers, anxious to begin teaching, should not at this point think that all that follows can be accomplished immediately. Typically, new teachers are most often concerned first with such things as the general ability level of their students, the kinds of materials available for teaching, or the grading practices usually employed. These and similar concerns are important and they should have priority right now.

There are several preparatory steps new teachers can take before scheduled teaching activities begin; most of them are appropriate, to varying degrees, in any setting in health science education. If they are taken at an early stage, the new teacher will be on a more even footing with experienced colleagues when beginning the first teaching experience.

During the process of gathering together materials that relate to a new course or unit of instruction, the teacher should take time to become familiar with any prerequisite courses or units that precede it. By talking to instructors of prerequisite courses, the new teacher can determine the content they present, how they present it, how they measure student achievement, and how they establish their standards or policies for grading.

Inquiries about recent student performance in colleagues' courses can reveal to what extent students have been meeting their course expectations. This is a good indication of how sound a foundation they have for subsequent courses. Asking about examination grade distributions or patterns of mistakes students have made in the past might serve to reveal content or skill areas that have caused difficulties. Some students coming into a new teacher's course after completing a biochemistry prerequisite, for example, may have experienced difficulty in applying either biological or chemical principles; neither difficulty would have been apparent in their final grades.

This kind of information unfortunately is not always automatically made available to new teachers—or to established teachers, for that matter. It is especially important, though, because it indicates the types of learning experiences students have had and thus the degree of preparation they are bringing to the new course. Knowledge of both can help guide the new teacher's own planning activities. While most instructors have never been asked to discuss this kind of information with colleagues, new teachers' experienced peers do so quite readily after interest has been expressed in what they are doing and in how it relates to someone else's teaching activities.

Just as new teachers should find out about the prerequisites for their own courses, they would also be well advised to find out which courses follow theirs in the curriculum. Getting to know the instructors of these courses, their expectations of students' entering skills, and what the instructors teach and how they do it can be just as helpful for planning one's own course as the information obtained about prerequisites. New teachers can broaden their perspectives by determining what is expected of their courses and the students completing them. Inquiring about other instructors' performance standards and the content, skills, behaviors, and abilities they expect students to possess can help a teacher formulate or solidify course goals and specific learning objectives.

When examining the teaching materials provided from previous offerings of a course or unit, teachers should first look for the overall goals and specific learning objectives that have been established. If these do exist, several questions should be asked: Are they precise and unambiguous? Do they correlate with what is now known about the course? Are they too general or excessively specific? The use of subjective judgment and the suggested formats for objectives discussed in subsequent chapters can help new teachers answer these questions.

If no objectives are available, or if existing objectives bear little resemblance to what the new teacher expects to be teaching, the next step is to look for a content outline. This should have been included with the course materials originally provided. If one exists, and if it appears to be up-to-date and comprehensive, it can provide a good source for an initial formulation of objectives. In the event an existing content outline is no longer entirely relevant, the necessary revisions can serve as natural stepping stones to the development of specific objectives. Revising or restructuring an existing content outline gives the new teacher a good understanding of the course or unit and what it should accomplish. Although this approach deviates from established educational procedures, such deviations are sometimes a practical necessity for new teachers who want to build a sound teaching program but must begin with limited, left-over materials.

Once existing objectives and outlines have been examined, revised, or reworked where necessary, the next step is to assess the quality and utility of the syllabus or schedule of teaching-learning activities used in the past. Is the given schedule easily followed, and does it logically lead the learner from the beginning to the end of the course or unit? Are the relationships among activities, resources, and deadlines clear? A syllabus or schedule of teaching-learning activities is as essential for a one-day nursing-skills workshop as it is for a semester-long course in periodontics.

Several elements should be referenced in a syllabus. For example, in the existing syllabus, have instructor presentations constituted the primary learning experiences available to students? Or have various other learning aids been incorporated? If other instructional methods, such as outside readings or slide-tapes, have been used before, how did they relate to the material covered? Where are the materials kept—on reserve, in the library, or in a learning re-source center? Is there any record of how effective they were? New teachers may discover some methods or tools through this process that they would feel comfortable including in their own course.

Media resources or self-instructional materials may have been used in the past; first assessments should involve their quality, their applicability to current instructional purposes, and their availability for future use. If such materials have not been used previously, arrangements can be made to preview new material. Most departments or schools have media or learning-materials centers, or have access to such units housed in a central library. Personnel in these units can assist in this phase of the inquiry. The same criteria used in judging textbooks and other printed teaching materials can be applied to media materials. These are: the existence of a direct relationship to the purpose, learning objectives, and content of a course; the teacher's own familiarity with the materials and their authors; and the costs to be borne by students and the department.

Just as new teachers should familiarize themselves with available teaching materials before beginning their teaching, they should also know the layout of the clinical, laboratory, or classroom facilities they will be using. While it is highly likely that they have worked previously in similar settings, it is still necessary for them to know how staffing configurations for teaching are scheduled, who provides support services, and who arranges student schedul-ing and provides for their materials or equipment in the new institution. Fur-ther, the nature and availability of teaching supplies and facilities should be ascertained. It would be futile, for example, to schedule media presentations if the assigned classroom lacked an appropriate seating arrangement, screen, or electrical outlets.

As the content to be taught and the methods for teaching it become clearer, a system of evaluation should be chosen that fits the identified objec-tives, is consistent and manageable, and will be understood and accepted by students. Different approaches to various types of evaluation are discussed in later chapters; the basic tenet of these discussions is that a successful evalua-tion program must be planned from the beginning along with and as part of one's teaching activities.

Finally, new teachers are given indications of personal and professional expectations during their position interviews and in subsequent communica-tions with department chairmen or supervisors. However, many of the details covered can easily be forgotten before teaching responsibilities actually begin, for not everything is included in written appointment letters, contracts, or agreements. After arriving on campus or assuming duties in an institution, it is therefore advisable to make sure a mutual understanding has been achieved concerning such things as the exact nature of teaching and professional responsibilities; the relative emphasis to be placed on nonteaching, service, and institutional activities; and the guidelines and criteria for professional advancement in the institution. A clarification of these and similar expectations at the beginning of a teaching career can help avoid frustration later on.

STAGES TO PASS THROUGH

As the first teaching experience draws near, what feelings might be anticipated? High levels of anxiety, a few sleepless nights, and the ever-present fear of failure should be expected, as well as the feeling of being overwhelmed by the new environment, demands, and deadlines. These are perfectly normal feelings, especially for the inexperienced teacher. Time and increased familiarity with the position will do much to diminish these insecurities.

New teachers should realize from the outset that they will never feel they have just taught the perfect course—something always seems to require revision or refinement. Even seasoned teachers, if they are effective, have recurrences of these same feelings. Such feelings do have a positive effect: they tend to keep teachers on their toes and actively involved in the teaching-learning process.

What happens next? The time for the first class finally arrives. Concerns about teaching that have been largely unconscious suddenly surface. They can contribute to fantasies of what might happen or what might go wrong in the classroom. A few restless nights are likely.

It can be a simple matter for new teachers to succumb to this rush of fantasies, to feel destined to fail. Again, a certain degree of anxiety is a natural accompaniment to any new or different undertaking and most teachers' fantasies are far worse than the reality of the classroom. It can be helpful to anticipate the upcoming teaching experience in terms of a framework describing the three stages of group life; this framework is discussed briefly here and in detail in Unit 3.

The first stage of group life involves developing a sense of trust between teacher and students. By allowing others to engage in "testing" behaviors and by consistently and fairly dealing with them in each testing situation, an individual can encourage trust in others.

The first few classes are characterized by a "honeymoon" period, during which neither teacher nor students have established a sense of mutual trust. Because students implicitly accord positions of authority to the teacher in a classroom, it is the teacher's responsibility to initiate and quickly cultivate a sense of trust with the students. By demonstrating an openness and honesty in the first class sessions, the teacher signals to students that a feeling of trust between them is indeed possible. This not only helps to create an environment conducive to learning, it also helps students proceed quickly through the testing phase in order to concentrate on their roles as learners in the course.

In the testing phase, students express in various indirect ways their concern about whether trust can be established. They may purposely ask questions for which the teacher has no ready answers, request a reiteration of something that has already been covered, or challenge the necessity of certain assignments. In each of these testing situations, the teacher should take care to adhere firmly to the guidelines and limits initially established and agreed on.

For example, if an assignment is being challenged, the teacher should not automatically assume that it is, in fact, a poor assignment. The students are testing to see if the teacher is firm, self-assured, and to be trusted. Likewise, in a situation where the teacher forgets or does not know something, it is best to be candid with the students. Such frankness helps them to see that they can be candid also. This is how, through testing, feelings of trust develop. At all costs, teachers should be direct and open with their students; hiding behind faculty rank, an institutional position, or a reputation as a clinician or scientist can only be destructive to teacher-student rapport.

When students have resolved their questions about the teacher, they stop testing and pass on into the second stage of group life, the working stage, where they begin serious work. This is the "good" part of the course.

The working stage, which is usually the middle portion of a course, is characterized by students knowing the expectations of the course and working hard to meet learning objectives. Teachers should therefore try to schedule the major elements of the course for the working stage. Because students are most productive at this stage, clinical, written, and outside projects are more meaningful if scheduled accordingly. Likewise, as much as possible, the bulk of the course should be presented midway—not overloaded at the beginning or saved until the end. Certainly there may be some tests or written papers that cannot be done until the last minute; however, this scheduling should be minimized as much as possible, since it does not support the normal life of the group and a well-developed group life has a definite influence on a teacher's effectiveness.

Lastly, from the very start, both teachers and students should anticipate and prepare for termination, the end or wrap-up stage. A course description that begins with a clear explication of objectives, an explanation of the amount of material students can expect to cover and the ways they can approach it, and a description of the amount of time the teacher has available for them paves the way for concluding the course. If, for example, a teacher is going to take a class for only six weeks of a semester, students should be told in advance, not at week four.

Groups end as they begin. New teachers can be fairly sure their students are terminating when they begin to engage in "testing" again. In fact, students may even ask the same questions about the course at the end as they did at the beginning. This should not be surprising, since activities such as parties and socializing usually mark both the beginning and end of a relationship. Some new behaviors may develop as well, such as denial that the course is over, anger over just getting good at a subject and then having to start fresh with another course, and perhaps even some depression that the course is at an end. New teachers should expect to experience similar feelings themselves towards their course and their students. These feelings help the teacher and students begin to separate, establish some distance between themselves, and prepare for termination of the course.

In sum, these are some of the feelings new teachers can anticipate, some of the behaviors to look for in a group of students, and the stages of group life they can expect to pass through in their first teaching experience. Each topic is discussed in more detail in later chapters. So as not to succumb to defensiveness in the actual teaching situation, new teachers should recognize that their anxiety level is bound to be very high at the beginning of a new course and that they are likely to feel, and indeed appear, awkward in front of their students. These are normal occurrences that diminish in frequency and intensity as the role of teacher becomes more familiar.

2
APPROACHING THE RESPONSIBILITIES OF TEACHING

As individuals assume the role of teacher in the health sciences, they assume responsibility for activities that will contribute to the preparation of health-care professionals. This responsibility is expressed through a variety of tasks and duties whose common purpose is to contribute to the effectiveness of professional education.

There are as many ways to meet the responsibilities of teaching as there are teachers. Individuals invariably bring to the teaching role their own personalities, character traits, strengths, and weaknesses, which are then tempered by the traditions of their institutions, the nature of their academic disciplines, and the type and extent of their teaching preparation.

Teachers in health science programs are members of the general community of a larger institution, whether they teach in a university school of pharmacy or a junior-college dental-assistant program. Because of this membership, new teachers tend to adopt the general approaches to teaching responsibilities that are sanctioned by their colleagues and their institution. These approaches, which are based more on tradition than on educational principles, are tempered in turn by the demands of specific professions.

New teachers in most health science programs are usually introduced to institutional routines and teaching practices by colleagues; these fellow teachers offer tips and suggestions collected over the course of years of experience. Such assistance tends to foster traditional approaches to education, for, by suggesting methods or techniques that new teachers experienced as students, seasoned colleagues attach a certain degree of credibility to them. Typically, new teachers react enthusiastically to these suggestions, relieved to have something concrete with which to face students. Ironically, they are incorporating many of the practices they themselves objected to as students.

Because it has often been assumed that a good health professional is automatically a good teacher, principles of teaching have not been an integral part of the professional preparation of those who teach in most of the health sciences. As a result, both the new teacher and the established teacher must rely largely on personal, in-service, or staff development efforts to develop competencies in this area. Such efforts could perhaps best be directed at developing an understanding of the nature of the teaching-learning process; a knowledge of the variety of activities, methods, techniques, and devices that can be used in it; and ultimately an ability to competently conduct the teaching-learning process.

APPROACHES TO TEACHING AND LEARNING

The overall goal of health science education programs is the preparation of new professionals able to manage their own behavior. Regardless of the profession or the situation, newly prepared health professionals must be able to utilize their personal resources to choose from alternatives, establish priorities, and problem solve as they contribute to the maintenance of health. Approaches to teaching and learning that are intended to prepare individuals to manage their own behavior as professionals should also encourage them to manage their own behavior as students.

Before adopting a specific approach to teaching and learning, and before selecting the activities, techniques, and methods that contribute to its formulation, a basic understanding of underlying assumptions and principles is needed if coherence and consistency are to characterize the teaching-learning process.

The Associationist Approach

There are two major approaches to the teaching-learning process. One of them has been developed by educators, psychologists, and researchers who are commonly identified as *associationists*. This group includes behaviorists, neobehaviorists, and connectionists.

Although they are concerned with different aspects of the teaching-learning process and differ somewhat as to specific emphases or methods, associationists basically agree that learning is a change in either verbal or nonverbal behaviors which occurs as the result of repetition. Their work is based largely on the assumption that learning takes place by students experiencing repeated associations between a stimulus and the correct response to it. While a particular stimulus can be directed at any of the senses, the response it is intended to evoke must be the same whenever the stimulus is given (6).

For students to learn in a particular subject area, the subject must first be broken down into a series of small units or stages. Each unit or stage itself is then divided into small pieces of information; through repetition and reinforcement, students learn the correct answers to questions about the small pieces of information. By continuing to respond correctly, students progress through the sequence of units or stages that make up a subject. Learning is thus largely the result of an accumulation of responses to various stimuli that have been arranged in some logical order (7).

Within the framework of the associationists, teaching is seen as arranging for appropriate conditions to expedite the required learning. The teacher decides which specific behaviors students are to exhibit and then provides the right stimuli at the right time, so that students in receiving roles will respond in the desired manner. This approach to teaching requires a *teacher-centered* classroom, for if students are to be successful, the teacher must be able to manage the various conditions for learning, manipulate appropriate stimuli or reinforcers, and ultimately control the behavior of students in the teaching-learning process.

Teachers who adopt a strictly associationist approach to teaching and learning construct their courses by first dividing the subject content to be taught into units made up of smaller steps or discrete bits of information. Lectures, discussions, or labs are then scheduled according to the sequence of steps established; their common purpose is to facilitate students' accomplishment of each step in the sequence.

Lectures present factual information related to specific steps of a unit; they are supplemented by readings in textbooks or journals. Student progress is evaluated through frequent quizzes on lecture material and reading assignments and through one or more major tests. In each instance the quiz or test is objective-based—e.g., made up of multiple-choice questions—and is quickly corrected and returned to students.

Discussions are scheduled at specific intervals to elaborate or clarify the information presented in lectures and the texts or journal articles. Through questioning, the teacher determines students' grasp of information and their readiness to proceed to new material. This setting thus provides the opportunity for teachers to work with small groups of students and to reinforce or modify their current behavior.

Laboratory work provides the opportunity for reinforcing students' responses to specific information by placing the information in a work situation that requires physical participation. The procedures, tasks, or experiments to be conducted are first set out in a step-by-step manner, with detailed instructions given by the teacher or contained in a workbook. Student performance is periodically assessed in the lab by the teacher, and the log or workbook kept by students is evaluated for accuracy once the lab period has ended.

In each of these instances, if a strictly associationist approach is taken, provision is made for personalized instruction, permitting students to proceed through the units and steps at their own pace. This provision necessarily implies the need for remedial material for slower students and supplementary material for advanced students.

The Cognitive Approach

The second major approach to teaching and learning, the *cognitive approach,* is advocated by the Gestalt-field and cognitive-field theorists. Other supporters of this approach are the proponents of discovery learning.

The cognitive approach views learning as a purposeful, goal-directed activity involving the gaining or changing of knowledge, skills, or abilities. It is based on the assumption that learning takes place by individuals reacting to, organizing, and then going beyond the information immediately related to a problem situation in order to develop new meanings for themselves. Learning is thus viewed as the result of resolving a problematical situation; in achieving this resolution, fundamental relationships, principles, or methods are understood and therefore made usable by the learner(4).

For students to learn in a particular subject area, problem solving on various levels takes place. Initially students confront problem situations that require only the application of previous knowledge for solution. As students progress through problem situations, and as their ability to problem solve develops, the nature of new problems gradually changes, so that previous knowledge alone is insufficient or inappropriate for their resolution. Students successfully solve new problems through inductive thinking, by which new principles or meanings are discovered and become usable (1).

Within the cognitive framework, teaching can be seen as creating an environment that promotes the problem-solving process; the teacher becomes a facilitator, assisting students through the process of induction as they engage in problem-solving activities. This approach to teaching requires a *student-centered* classroom, for successful problem solving is a highly individualistic and self-directed process. It requires that each student examine a problem situation and organize information and experience according to a personal cognitive framework.

Teachers who adopt a strictly cognitive approach to teaching and learning establish their courses by first identifying the range of problem situations inherent in particular subject content and then by guiding students individually through the induction process, so that various levels of problem solving can be attained.

Because of the highly individualistic nature of this type of learning, emphasis is placed on learning activities that encourage individual participation. Lectures or large-group presentations are minimized, if not omitted entirely. If employed, they are used to reiterate prerequisite information, principles, or methods each student should have, or to present new problem situations to students assembled as a group.

Small-group discussions are the major means for student-teacher interaction on a group basis. Rather than being teacher-directed, these sessions are conducted by students who raise, discuss, and answer questions of each other, utilizing the teacher as a resource and guide when needed. As an extension of these sessions, each student pursues a project or investigation independently of the others; this project could relate to one or a series of problem situations raised in group presentations. Structured laboratory work as such is not scheduled; rather, laboratory time is provided for interested students as one means for conducting their own investigations.

Evaluation of student progress is based on the teacher's review of each student's analytic performance in the small-group setting; on written examinations constructed to test problem-solving abilities; and on an assessment of each student's investigatory project, both in terms of the process and the product it represents.

These admittedly brief summaries of the two major approaches to teaching and learning are intended only to highlight the need for teachers to begin to develop an understanding of the assumptions and principles underlying various facets of the teaching-learning process. Reaching at least a basic understanding can contribute ultimately to the coherence and consistency of an individual teacher's activities in the classroom.

It is beyond present purposes to further discuss the various elements of major approaches to teaching and learning, or to relate the research conducted in these areas to health science education. For those interested in delving further, references have been included in the Unit 1 bibliography to provide a starting point for independent inquiries.

As their inquiries progress, both new teachers and experienced teachers generally find they are unable to adopt exclusively or implement fully one approach in classroom practice. For example, while there is an abundance of research describing the effectiveness of such applications of stimulus-response principles as computer-assisted instruction and programmed textbooks, the question is still open as to whether such techniques by themselves can promote or lead to problem solving. Further, although the process and product of each student's problem solving will be unique and highly personal, the level of difficulty and time commitment associated with this approach make it all but impossible to develop for a large group of students working under the constraints of an institutional time schedule.

It is therefore quite possible that teachers' inquiries will lead to eclectic selections of methods and techniques based on their particular needs. This is a workable procedure, chosen also for the development of this book, since many elements of the major approaches are not incompatible. Selection criteria should evolve from the purposes of a particular educational program, the resources and constraints inherent in the program, and the desire to encourage students to develop in the teaching-learning process the same competencies they will need as professionals.

COMPONENTS OF TEACHING

A traditional approach to teaching in the health sciences has teachers assuming the role of fact giver and students assuming the complementary role of passive receiver of information. An alternative approach, appropriate to the overall goals of health science education programs, views teachers and students as participants in a teaching-learning transaction, a multifaceted agreement to work together toward the goals of a specific course.

Before entering into a transaction with students, the teacher's initial responsibility is to create an environment that will promote different kinds and different levels of student learning. This environment is fostered by the way teaching is developed—i.e., by the way activities, methods, strategies, and materials together constitute the approach a teacher and students take in pursuing a course of study. An overall approach to organizing and conducting teaching activities that encourages a transaction between teachers and students and that capitalizes on their respective roles in the teaching-learning process can be based on these four interdependent stages:

1. *Planning:* the identification of the goals of teaching and of the personal and material resources needed to assist students in achieving those goals.
2. *Development:* the preparation of the personal and material elements required for teaching.
3. *Management:* the execution of teaching activities; the manner in which transactions between teachers and students take place.
4. *Evaluation:* the assessment of the effectiveness of the process and the product of teaching.

The basic relationship of these stages is depicted in Fig. 2.1. Planning forms the basis for all other teaching activities; development entails gathering together the various resources identified as essential for managing teaching activities; management brings together planning and development activities in teaching-learning transactions; and evaluation provides the means for determining the effectiveness of the process and its products and for beginning the process once again. Depending on specific contexts of time and purpose, as is described in subsequent chapters, some activities of the various stages can occur either simultaneously or in somewhat altered sequences.

This four-stage approach to teaching can be applied to teacher activities at the course level—for example, in planning a six-week course in chemotherapy—and to those at the specific activity level—for example, in producing

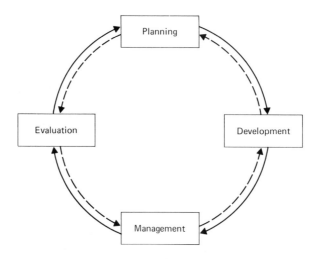

Fig. 2.1
Relationship of four stages of an overall approach
to organizing and conducting teaching activities.

a slide-tape program on characteristics of malignant cell behavior. This approach is also appropriate for general curriculum development, although this aspect is not formally treated here.

Planning

The Planning Stage

Identify/state goals and objectives.
Select subject content.
Sequence subject content.
Identify resources and constraints.
Allocate instructional time.
Select instructional methods and materials.
Develop an evaluation plan.
Assess student characteristics.

Activities of the planning stage vary in emphases according to the teacher's purpose, time, and subject-content requirements. While the specification of objectives is the necessary first step in planning to teach, there is no inherent sequence that must be followed for the other activities. If, for example, a new course with an unfamiliar group of students is to be conducted, a step-by-step approach through the activities is probably needed. If, on the other hand, a course previously taught is being refined, undoubtedly more emphasis should be placed on some of the activities, such as selecting new instructional methods, and less on others, such as selecting and sequencing subject content.

The first component of the planning stage is *stating instructional goals and specific learning objectives.* An instructional goal is a generalized statement of intent, a description of an anticipated end or outcome of instruction. It indicates the purpose of teaching and, at the same time, identifies its relationship to the overall purposes of the curriculum or preparation program (3). Teachers, by stating instructional goals from their vantage points as content resource persons and professionals in specific fields, indicate for themselves, their students, and their colleagues what they expect can be accomplished in the teaching-learning process. The following instructional goals from a teaching unit on infectious diseases illustrate the general nature of goals:

- Understands the principles of the host-parasite interrelationship.
- Knows the relationship of infectious diseases to nonsuppurative complications, such as chronic bronchitis or rheumatic fever.
- Applies the principles of detection and control of infections to given clinical case studies.

The teaching-learning process is goal directed; it is directed at the attainment of the instructional goals identified for a course of study. Specific learning objectives provide a detailed approach to the overall goals; they indicate in precise terms the knowledge, skills, or abilities students should develop in order to effectively accomplish the goals of the teaching-learning process (3).

Specific learning objectives become the criteria for evaluating student achievement as successful or unsuccessful. They are therefore stated in performance terms that can be measured and evaluated, as are the following objectives, developed for a section on infectious mononucleosis:

- Performs commercial latex slide agglutination tests.
- Performs presumptive tube tests for heterophile antibody.
- Interprets agglutination and hemolysis patterns.
- Correlates lab test results with clinical findings.

The process of stating instructional goals and specific learning objectives is the essential first activity in the planning sequence, for its results provide teachers with a guide for the rest of their instructional activities. (They later also provide students with a guide for their learning activities.) The initial statement of objectives, for example, forms the framework for the second activity of the planning stage, *selecting subject content.*

Subject content is that which has been learned about a subject—the entire store of theories, principles, relationships, and facts amassed over time by study of the subject. Although teachers begin their planning with an overall conception of the subject content they will be teaching, the statements of objectives serve to identify specific content areas for a course of study. In essence, this is a sampling process; teachers must select from a subject's store of knowledge only that content students need to acquire to achieve specific learning objectives.

Closely associated with selecting subject content is the third activity included in the planning stage, *sequencing subject content*. The primary purpose in sequencing content is to provide a continuous, integrated approach to a subject. Thus the process of sequencing is conducted in terms of what and how students should learn in order to achieve course objectives, rather than solely in terms of what teachers and their colleagues know about the subject.

A plan or framework for sequencing can reflect one or more dimensions of the logical relationships between and among natural divisions, subdivisions, or boundaries of the subject itself. It can also be influenced by an institution's curricular design requirements, which may identify specific emphases for subject content in individual courses. There is no single correct sequence; whichever plan for sequencing is found to be most appropriate and most helpful should be used in the context of the goals and objectives established so far.

After content has been selected and sequenced, the teacher can begin *identifying resources and constraints* and *allocating instructional time to subject content*. By identifying resources available for instruction, teachers determine which methods, materials, or facilities they will or will not be able to include in the teaching-learning process. The ready availability of audiotapes on auscultation and heart sounds in a physical-diagnosis course, for example, could free the teacher to work with students on inspecting and palpating the anterior chest after the students had worked independently with the media units.

The identification of constraints—those conditions or situations that limit a teacher's flexibility—also contributes to the way a course is eventually carried out. Assignment to a large lecture hall, for example, necessarily limits the type and quality of class discussion possible. The development of a course and the way subject content is to be covered can also be restricted by institutional time schedules (length of class period, teaching day, or term); by the financial support the institution provides for teaching; and by the relative availability of equipment.

Instructional time refers to specific time commitments required by the various elements that contribute to the teaching-learning process. It can be allocated according to the way that process is developed, e.g., according to specific content emphases, teaching methods, or resources and constraints. Allocating instructional time can also be guided by the nature of specific content divisions or areas: some are prerequisites to others and thus need sufficient emphasis to ensure that students are ready to go on; others supplement major topics and can be covered by students on an individual basis.

Once again, the basic guide for allocating instructional time should be the established learning objectives. The relative amount of time spent on specific content areas and specific activities should directly assist students in achieving those objectives.

Identifying resources and constraints and allocating instructional time are also closely associated with a sixth activity included in the planning stage, *selecting instructional methods and materials.* Instructional methods describe how teachers participate in the teaching-learning process, while instructional materials are the tools and devices used to support and augment their participation. The traditional method of health science education has been the lecture; the traditional materials have been printed handouts and reading assignments. Although both have their advantages, many other effective methods and materials exist. (Many of these methods and materials are treated in later chapters.)

A seventh activity in the planning stage, *developing an evaluation plan*, is based on decisions concerning the assessment of student learning—i.e., the knowledge, skills, or abilities that indicate the level of a student's achievement of specific learning objectives. This activity is also based on decisions concerning the assessment of the effectiveness of the teaching-learning process. Both kinds of decisions involve identifying elements that are measurable; selecting procedures and devices that can be used to obtain effective and efficient measures; and establishing standards to be used in interpreting the results of evaluation activities.

Evaluation decisions often are postponed indefinitely, until the need for some kind of assessment process can no longer be ignored. This is in part due to a certain uneasiness many teachers experience with evaluation activities and to the common misconception that evaluation is sequentially the last thing to be done in teaching. Incorporating evaluation with other planning activities not only enhances the validity and reliability of evaluation mechanisms, it also contributes to overall decision making as a teaching program is developed.

The last activity included in the planning stage, *assessing student characteristics*, forms a bridge between the planning and management stages of instruction. By assessing student characteristics at the start of instruction, teachers are essentially performing a task similar to taking a patient history at the start of medical intervention. A knowledge of students' characteristics, such as the extent of their entering knowledge of the subject content of the course, their individual preferences for methods of learning, and their own objectives for enrolling in the course, helps to define the direction instruction will take. This permits both teacher and students to make optimal use of the time they have together.

Assessing individual and group student characteristics can also contribute to the sense of trust that must be established between teacher and students. By conducting an assessment, a teacher communicates concern for the individuality of students. Efforts to use the results of such an assessment, even if they fall short of original intentions, indicate the teacher's interest in developing worthwhile transactions with students.

Development

The Development Stage

Arrange course schedule.
Sequence learning experiences.
Prepare instructional materials.
Prepare lectures, labs, etc.

The development stage entails activities with a curricular focus, those that take place prior to instruction and represent an extension of planning activities; and activities with an instructional focus, those that take place during or as a result of instruction.

Development activities with a curricular focus can include writing a course outline, preparing handouts, or establishing a time schedule of class meetings, readings, assignments, and related learning experiences. These activities, which together constitute constructing a syllabus, form the curricular framework for the teaching-learning process.

Development activities leading to the construction of a syllabus represent the first steps in implementing the teaching plans so far established. Once content has been selected and sequenced, time allocated to content and to instructional activities, and resources and constraints identified, the teacher can begin *arranging a time schedule of course or class meetings*. This schedule includes the times and dates of the various types of class sessions, such as lectures, discussions, or clinical experiences. It reflects the course objectives, subject content, and the time framework of the institution.

As this schedule is arranged, the instructional goals and specific learning objectives are written out in final form, the latter divided by content sequence or other divisional framework used to mark the parts of the course. Included along with the specific learning objectives is the content outline; it can take the form of key words or phrases placed alongside the objectives, or it can be a separate, more extensive discussion of major content areas. Either way, the specific learning objectives and the content outline together serve as the essential curricular framework for both teacher and students.

Another step in the development process, one that involves filling out this initial framework, is *establishing the sequence of readings, assignments, or other learning experiences*. The elements of this sequence are used by students in working to achieve specific learning objectives and come from the texts, references, and resources already identified for the course. Readings, assignments, or other learning experiences, such as group problem-solving sessions, can complement and supplement the teaching-learning process as it evolves.

If learning packages, gaming activities, or media materials are to be incorporated in the teaching-learning process, and the commercial materials that were previewed seem to be inadequate, another development activity, *preparing instructional materials,* is necessary. The preparation of any instructional material, whether a learning package or a videotape, follows similar basic steps: (1) identify and write learning objectives for the new resource; (2) select and sequence the content of the new resource; (3) arrange for its production; (4) incorporate the resource in the teaching-learning process; and (5) evaluate its effectiveness as a teaching device.

Certain other development activities occur during the teaching-learning process or as a result of the process. They can include *preparing lecture presentations, discussions, laboratory or clinical activities, or personalized instructional activities.* These activities reflect a certain flexibility on the part of the teacher, for while they follow the basic developmental sequence just outlined, they are also particularly affected by the characteristics of students in the course, their idiosyncratic interests, skills, and abilities.

The initial assessment of student characteristics provides the basis for the direction to be taken in a course of study. Subsequent assessments made through either objective measurements, subjective observations, or both, further describe the students enrolled. Thus, while preparation of laboratory activities necessarily must occur before students engage in them, this preparation is guided by recent experiences with students in the teaching-learning process. Similarly, while provisions must be made in advance for contingency contracting (a written agreement whose outcome is dependent on student performance of the terms of the agreement), the development of the contract is a function of prior instruction, of what a teacher knows about the students who wish to enter into a contract, and of the manner in which particular students accept the objectives of the course. In other words, the teacher should be prepared for a variety of types of students.

Development activities, then, whether of a curricular or instructional focus, provide the bridge between the planning of instruction and the management of specific plans.

Management

The Management Stage

Lecture.
Lead seminars/discussions.
Conduct laboratory experiences.
Conduct clinical experiences.
Arrange for personalized instruction.
Refine teaching skills.

The management stage encompasses those teaching activities that bring together planning and development efforts as teachers transact with students.

The teaching-learning process in health science education has usually taken place in four traditional forms: lecture presentation, seminar/discussion, clinical experience, and laboratory experience. Each of these forms includes the techniques, devices, or materials arranged for in previous stages and each requires, to differing degrees, the use of common skills, such as working with groups, managing learning problems, and motivating students.

By *lecturing*, the teacher assumes a directive role to convey a structured body of knowledge to a group of students. The teacher transmits to students knowledge they do not have or would have difficulty, as novices, obtaining on their own. The lecture draws together diverse subject-content elements in order to assist students in developing understandings, insights, or relationships needed to achieve the learning objectives of a course.

Although the lecture presentation requires the transmission of knowledge to students, it does not mean students are passive or noninvolved. Indeed, the most successful lecturers are those who encourage active participation by students. This participation can easily occur in small to moderate-sized groups and can include critique periods, continual feedback during lecture, the solicitation of examples or illustrations, or the acceptance of responses to questions or problems related to the content of the lecture (5).

By *leading seminar/discussions*, the teacher engages in cooperative problem solving, an exchange of ideas, or a logical dialogue with students. In leading a discussion with students, the major purpose is threefold. The teacher strives to assist them in approaching an issue, problem, or situation; in identifying and analyzing various points of view or research findings; and in arriving at some conclusions, resolutions, or positions for themselves. The discussion process thus requires active student involvement. It should encourage them to express their own positions, to think in terms of the subject content being discussed, and to develop skill in formulating and expressing ideas as well as in listening to others do the same.

Like the lecture, the discussion frequently suffers from teacher misuse, primarily inadequate teacher preparation. Regardless of the academic level of students, some individuals in each class are bound to have difficulty expressing themselves, either because they lack appropriate verbal skills or because they are unwilling or unable to make a substantive contribution to the discussion. Further, the natural diversity in most student groups can be exacerbated by varying levels of student preparation for a discussion. Thus, it is essential that teachers not only possess group skills, but also have some understanding of the abilities and characteristics of their students. It is also essential that they identify and communicate to students in advance of the discussion which topic, issue, or problem is to be covered, as well as which readings, materials, or media are requisite for their participation.

By *conducting the laboratory experience*, the teacher provides the means for students to confront and apply facts, principles, and relationships of subject content in a practical, working environment. The laboratory experience complements the lecture presentation, discussion, or independent study by giving students an opportunity to apply the information presented to them.

The laboratory experience, whether for anatomy, pharmaceutics, or immunology, affords an excellent opportunity for problem-solving activities. Like the lecture and discussion, the laboratory experience brings together information, principles, and concepts as students dissect, experiment, or perform test procedures. Thus, like other problem-solving activities, the laboratory experience requires presession preparation by students; an initial clarification of the problem, procedure, or test to be approached in the session; and close monitoring of individual students as each progresses to a conclusion or resolution.

By *conducting the clinical experience*, the teacher provides the means for students to begin their professional contacts with patients and to encounter firsthand real patient problems requiring immediate solution. Like the laboratory experience, the clinical experience complements other teaching-learning activities. To varying degrees, students are able to apply to actual patient-care situations knowledge previously learned. Unlike the laboratory experience, which is largely controlled or structured, the clinical experience very often presents unanticipated conditions or situations and requires information, skills, or abilities students may not yet have mastered. As a learning resource, it is therefore perhaps the most valuable and effective problem-solving or decision-making activity for students.

The first phase of managing teaching activities involves providing for the general needs of all students. This is usually accomplished in the health sciences through some combination of lecture, discussion, laboratory, or clinical experience. The second phase involves providing for the variety of individual backgrounds, interests, or abilities of the students. This can be accomplished through such strategies as independent study or contingency contracting. Both strategies entail *personalizing the teaching-learning process,* so that a one-to-one relationship between teacher and student is achieved.

Both forms of personalized instruction are based on providing alternate pathways for students of differing abilities or interests to work toward the goals of a course of study. Pathways may be designed for slower students with some identified learning problem; for gifted students who have the ability to learn faster than the average student; for students whose interests and personal objectives diverge from those of their peers; and for students whose preferences for learning cannot easily be addressed by the scheduled teaching-learning process.

As part of the management process, teachers should be concerned with *refining their skills in leading groups, motivating learners, and managing learning problems.* Teachers often have expertise in one or more of these areas, simply because of their life experiences, previous courses, or academic experiences. The difficulty lies in applying the skills or knowledge they have gained elsewhere to teaching in the health sciences. Group skills can be approached in terms of the three phases of group life and the role of the teacher in each phase, and in terms of common group problems, such as silence, anger, and testing. Factors that affect motivation can be approached through emphasis on encouraging interest in learning. These, in turn, relate to specific learning problems, such as the slow learner, the immature learner, and the gifted learner, and require attention to the role of the teacher in managing these learning problems.

The management of the teaching-learning process, then, can occur in a variety of ways, each of which represents the culmination of planning and development activities expressed as actual transactions with students.

Evaluation

The Evaluation Stage

Assess student learning.
Assess teaching-learning process.

The last stage of teaching, evaluation, provides the means for determining the effectiveness of the previous stages. Evaluation should not be viewed as an activity that occurs only once at the end of a course of study, but as a dynamic process that can provide continuous feedback to both teachers and students.

There are three phases to any evaluation activity: examination, diagnosis, and prescription. Examination refers to the process of gathering and recording data and requires that decisions be made concerning what should be evaluated, when it should be evaluated, and how the evaluation should be conducted. Diagnosis refers to the process of utilizing the data obtained through the examination phase and involves making decisions in light of the criteria or standards established for the evaluation activity. Prescription refers to the process of taking appropriate action in response to the evaluation results. The nature of these phases makes it essential that evaluation be considered an integral part of all stages of teaching if it is to be effective and useful.

Evaluation is conducted for the purpose of *assessing student learning* in a course of study, whether that learning takes place in a classroom, laboratory, or clinical setting.

Like many other facets of teaching, evaluation activities are affected by considerations of time, available resources, and practicality. Further, because learning is a complex, multifaceted process, with complex, multifaceted results, any device to measure it can at best measure only a representative sample of all possible content areas and specific learning objectives (2).

Evaluation is also conducted for the purpose of *assessing the effectiveness of the teaching-learning process*. While the ultimate measure of effectiveness is the degree to which students have achieved learning objectives, the nature of the contribution the teacher makes to that achievement should also be identified and assessed. Further, the printed and media materials that are used, the facilities and resources that are available, and the variety of devices incorporated in the teaching-learning process all have an influence on the effectiveness of the process and thus on the nature of student learning. Hence, a teacher's planning, development, and management activities are evaluated as they combine to form the teacher's transactions with students.

Any evaluation effort should be anticipated and arranged for in the planning stage and referenced directly to teachers' ultimate criteria—that is, their instructional goals and specific learning objectives. The results of evaluation then become the basis for subsequent planning, development, and management activities as teaching is revised and refined.

A RECAPITULATION

The four stages that make up an approach to teaching, along with their constituent activities, are depicted in Fig. 2.2.

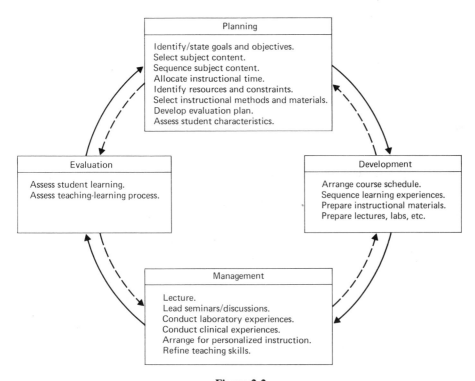

Figure 2.2

The first step to be taken in this approach—identifying and stating instructional goals and specific learning objectives—becomes the skeletal framework for all subsequent steps and activities. It also provides the ultimate criteria for judging the process and the product of teaching.

The emphasis given to specific activities in each stage of the approach will vary according to the teacher's expertise and familiarity with the course material. A new teacher responsible for a new course of study will probably place equal emphasis on as many specific activities as possible, in order to lay the foundation for effective teaching. With the experience of teaching a particular course at least once comes the ability to identify areas that need more emphasis than others. Further, the experienced teacher will find that many of the activities of this four-stage approach begin to assume a carry-over quality; for example, an effective slide-tape program can be used several times a course is taught, rather than developing a new one each time, just as a simulation evaluation exercise can be used with more than one group of students.

The primary purpose of this four-stage framework is to provide health science teachers with a systematic, straightforward approach to carrying out their own teaching responsibilities. The approach is intended to help teachers effectively engage in transactions with their students, transactions that will permit both teacher and student to realize their potential roles in the teaching-learning process.

REFERENCES

1. BAYLES, ERNEST E. *The Theory and Practice of Teaching.* New York: Harper & Row, 1950.
2. GRONLUND, NORMAN E. *Measurement and Evaluation in Teaching.* 2d ed. New York: MacMillan, 1971.
3. GRONLUND, NORMAN E. *Stating Behavioral Objectives for Classroom Instruction.* New York: Macmillan, 1970.
4. HILGARD, ERNEST R., AND GORDON H. BOWER. *Theories of Learning.* 3d ed. New York: Appleton-Century-Crofts, 1966.
5. HYMAN, RONALD T. *Ways of Teaching.* Philadelphia: Lippincott, 1970.
6. LOGAN, FRANK A. *Fundamentals of Learning and Motivation.* Boston: Little, Brown, 1970.
7. SKINNER, B. F. *The Technology of Teaching.* New York: Appleton-Century-Crofts, 1968.

UNIT 1
THE PLANNING PROCESS

As individuals assume the role of teacher in the health sciences, they assume the responsibility of planning teaching activities that will contribute to the preparation of health-care professionals. This responsibility is expressed through a variety of tasks and duties whose common purpose is to assure the effectiveness of the teaching-learning process. The way teachers approach this responsibility, and the way they approach the performance of their teaching role, is ultimately based on their view of students and students' roles in the teaching-learning process.

The traditional view of students suggests that they are the passive recipients of knowledge generated or gathered together by a professional expert charged with teaching them. Teachers who adhere to this view thus approach the planning process with one primary objective in mind: to structure class-related activities so as to ensure efficient communication from teacher to students. On the other hand, if students are viewed as active, mature, pre-professional individuals, a quite different approach to planning is required, one that ultimately permits them to develop and express themselves as individual learners in the teaching-learning process.

Teachers should be aware that the way they view students can become a self-fulfilling prophecy, especially when this view shapes their selection of teaching activities. Just as their approach to teaching dictates their own contributions to the teaching-learning process, so too does it implicitly determine a set of requirements for student learning. As a result, students assume either dependent or active roles in the teaching-learning process, depending on which they perceive is essential for success.

Students should be responsible for their own learning, just as they will shortly become responsible for their own professional behavior. Thus, the goal of the following approach to planning is to provide students the opportunity to participate actively in the teaching-learning process. This approach is discussed in the two chapters of Unit 1. Chapter 3 details the various activities comprising the planning stage and Chapter 4 considers different approaches teachers can take to assess learner characteristics and to relate the results of such an assessment to development activities.

3
PLANNING
TO TEACH

Systematic planning forms the foundation for any teaching. The way in which specific planning activities are conducted reflects the strengths and weaknesses, experience, abilities, and interests of individual teachers preparing for personal transactions with students.

While planning activities and the transactions they lead to are necessarily individualistic, they cannot be carried out in a vacuum. If appropriate teaching-learning transactions are to take place, teachers' planning must proceed within the framework of the professional education program established by the faculty. A description of the program indicates the type of abilities, skills, and attitudes a professional graduating from the program is expected to possess.

The curriculum established for this professional preparation is identified by its various components—e.g., its basic science, laboratory, or clinical components; their interrelationships; and their relationships to the behavior and activities of practicing professionals. Specific courses are then identified by their general instructional goals, their relationship to the purposes of the curriculum, and a summary of the content they address.

On a periodic basis the faculty, representative practitioners, students, and nonpractitioners should meet to review the purposes of the educational program and the structure and content of its curriculum. This review can be based on observed current health needs of the local and extended community; the continuing and projected needs of the community, outside agencies, and the health-care system itself; and the identified educational needs of current practitioners (7). These factors can help focus the review on detecting any existing gaps in the curriculum and curricular offerings, as well as current strengths and weaknesses. The ultimate result of the review would be a set of recommendations for refinement or revision of the educational program. These recommendations serve to respecify the purposes and content of an educational program. They also form the basis for individual teachers' development of instructional goals and specific learning objectives for their own courses, as well as the basis for the rest of their planning activities.

GOALS AND OBJECTIVES

General goals, instructional goals, major objectives, overall objectives, enabling objectives, specific learning objectives—new teachers and teachers unfamiliar with the seemingly arbitrary and often confusing nomenclature of educational jargon are sure to encounter difficulty and experience frustration when first attempting to state the purposes of their teaching. Their confusion is understandable, for are not goals and objectives the same thing? They are in common usage; but in teaching it is generally useful to distinguish between types or levels of goals and objectives.

A systematic approach to course construction and curriculum building entails identifying instructional goals and specific learning objectives.

Instructional Goals

Instructional goals represent what the teacher as a practitioner/clinician /subject-matter specialist feels students should derive from a course as a whole. Alternatively, instructional goals represent what students can expect from taking a course. Because they indicate the major purposes of a particular course, goals provide the general direction for planning, developing, managing, and evaluating a course (4).

Instructional goals relate a course to the curriculum for which it is being constructed. They serve to identify the parameters of subject content in terms of how much a particular subject can or should be covered (e.g., a biochemistry course that is part of the science component of a nursing curriculum has different parameters than one intended for biochemistry majors), and in terms of the level of students for which the course is intended (e.g., entering level, upper-division level, postgraduate level). They can also indicate the relationship of the course to others dealing with similar content. A "core" or basic course, for example, should reflect the fact that it provides a foundation for subsequent courses in the curriculum.

Goals can be derived from a variety of sources. Teachers charged with constructing a new course or with revising an existing one can begin the goal-setting process by considering the course's position in the total curriculum and in the sequence of courses dealing with related subject matter. Is the course intended to provide a foundation for subsequent courses? Does it represent the most extensive academic experience available in the curriculum for a particular content area? How should it relate to other courses, clinical experiences, or laboratory work that students will be involved in concurrently? These questions, when raised in terms of the results of a curriculum review, should begin to bring into focus the student needs that can be fulfilled by the course. In essence, then, the instructional goals of a course are developed through a question-and-answer process intended to define the course's major purposes, both short-term and long-term.

Goals are not easily measurable. For example, the instructional goals of a psychiatry course in an undergraduate medical curriculum could be:

- Appreciates the mental-health needs of patients.
- Understands the major psychiatric disorders in light of their history, epidemiology, and presumed etiologies.
- Performs basic diagnostic skills.
- Develops the ability to recognize patients' psychiatric needs in a non-psychiatric medical setting.

The first goal listed would obviously be quite difficult to break down into quantifiable parts and measure on a final exam. The second lends itself to measurement by forming the basis for further, specific objectives for individual units of the course; the third possesses similar characteristics. The fourth is much like the first, essential to the character of the course, but not easily measurable because of its long-range implications. All goals, however, provide the general direction for the way the course is planned, developed, managed, and evaluated.

Learning Objectives

Once teachers have decided with some certainty what their instructional goals should be, the development of specific learning objectives takes place. Learning objectives serve two basic purposes: they represent what students should be able to do in each content area or unit of a course and, taken together, they direct students' achievement of the instructional goals established for the course (4). While instructional goals by their nature are not easily amenable to measurement, specific learning objectives are; they become the criteria for evaluating student performance.

There are two kinds of specific learning objectives. They reflect different levels of teaching and learning and, therefore, carry different implications for subsequent course-construction activities. They are referred to as "minimal competence" and "developmental competence" objectives.

Mimimal competence objectives These objectives focus on specific aspects of behavior—i.e., some knowledge, skill, or ability—that all students are expected to develop. They indicate a minimal level of performance to be attained and therefore usually function as prerequisites to further learning in a specific content area.

These objectives, the methods of learning and instructional procedures they suggest, and the techniques for evaluating their achievement are best matched with the associationist approach to the teaching-learning process (see Chapter 2). As discussed earlier, the associationist approach views learning as a stimulus-response activity. Minimal competence objectives, by their very nature, can best be achieved through such an approach. Consider the following minimal competence objectives, included in a cardiovascular unit in an introductory physiology course:

- States proper units for designating blood flow.
- Identifies pressure-volume changes during each period of the cardiac cycle.
- Correlates the waves of lead II of the electrocardiogram with the conduction of the cardiac impulse.

Each of these objectives, while focusing on different concepts or principles, represents facets of cardiovascular physiology that students would be expected to master to be minimally competent in the area. The first objective, for example, represents a specific, low-level behavior students would be required to possess before starting a section on hemodynamics. The second objective represents a somewhat higher level of performance than the first; it requires previous knowledge of volume and pressure principles as a prelude to the study of the four phases of the cardiac cycle. The third objective also represents a higher level of performance than the first; it requires students to associate previous knowledge of the origin and conduction of the cardiac impulse to recording methods and lead arrangements of the electrocardiogram. Achievement of this objective would necessarily be requisite to later laboratory work.

While indicative of different topics and somewhat different abilities, the three objectives are all characterized by the fact that (1) the students' task is clearly identified prior to any instruction, (2) the teacher prepares appropriate visual materials or handouts which may accompany a lecture presentation of the content related to each objective, and (3) the students are tested on their ability to perform the tasks specified in the objectives. Because specific items test behaviors reflecting basic performance levels, it is expected that each student be able to answer each item correctly (5).

Developmental competence objectives These objectives focus on aspects of behavior that should be developed by students to differing degrees, depending on their respective abilities and performance capabilities. Because they indicate levels of performance beyond the minimal competence level, complete attainment by all students is not expected. Therefore, they usually serve to delineate advanced learning in a specific content area.

While minimal competence objectives represent single behaviors, developmental competence objectives do not. They typically call for complex behaviors on the part of students, for example, to be able to understand, analyze, interpret, or apply. These types of abilities take time to develop, so each student should be encouraged to pursue them to the maximum extent possible in a particular course. They differ from minimal competence objectives in that they are more open-ended; they do not end with demonstration of a basic proficiency.

Developmental competence objectives, the teaching and learning methods they suggest, and the techniques for evaluating their achievement by students are best matched with the cognitive approach to the teaching-learning process. Attainment of developmental competence objective involves a discovery or problem-solving process which students engage in with guidance from the teacher. This process can be illustrated by the following developmental competence objectives, included in the cardiovascular physiology unit mentioned earlier:

- *Example 1:* Explains the physiologic basis for the treatment of essential hypertension.
    1. Describes clinical manifestations of essential hypertension.
    2. Identifies inhibiting factors of the medullary vasomotor center.
    3. Describes changes in glomerular filtration in hypertensive conditions.

- *Example 2:* Analyzes the physiologic changes occurring in a simulated patient undergoing hemorrhagic shock.

Both objectives direct students to engage in a series of problem-solving activities in which they apply physiological principles to clinical situations. Students could work independently or in small groups, with assistance from the teacher when needed. The objectives therefore not only serve to encourage advanced study by students, they also function in this course as bridges between basic-science-oriented and clinical-oriented work.

The two objectives are written in slightly different formats. The objective in the first example is accompanied by abilities or behaviors that represent the developmental process to be followed in attaining the objective. Because they are samples of behaviors involved in developing an understanding of the physiological bases of hypertension treatment, they are not taught and tested on a one-to-one basis, but rather provide direction for the teaching-learning process. The objective in the second example does not include representative samples of behaviors related to an analysis of physiological changes. This format instead assumes that an appropriate series of objectives and content has preceded the objective. That these are both developmental competence objectives would be substantiated by the learning activities associated with them.

Because developmental competence objectives cannot be taught and tested on a one-to-one basis, and because they represent complex knowledge, skills, or abilities that individual students work toward to the maximum extent possible, evaluation mechanisms developed to measure their achievement necessarily identify differences in student performance (2). Essay examinations, projects, or simulation exercises are logical choices for measuring performance of this nature. Multiple-choice questions related to case studies, clinical situations, or laboratory studies can, with care, also be developed to measure the types of problem-solving called for by these objectives.

Various techniques and styles for stating objectives are available in the educational literature. Instead of repeating them here, the techniques and styles most appropriate to the concept of minimal and developmental competence objectives are referenced in the Unit 1 bibliography.

SELECTING SUBJECT CONTENT

The selection of specific subject content to include in a course is a sampling process, in which a teacher, after considering the whole subject and its constituent parts, chooses only that content students should confront to be able to achieve the specific learning objectives of the course.

The selection process rests on the assumption that a teacher is not only knowledgeable in a specific subject area, but also possesses an understanding of the basic logic of the subject. This logic includes the system of principles, relationships, and interrelationships underlying the facts, definitions, and analytic elements of a subject; it also includes the methods of verification employed in the subject, such as the manner in which new hypotheses are tested or the applicability of tested data is established (8).

A basic approach to selecting subject content for teachers knowledgeable in a specific subject involves referring to the curriculum review that has been conducted and examining the natural or traditional organization of the subject.

A schoolwide, divisional, or departmental curriculum review should identify stages of professional growth that students pass through on their way to becoming health-care professionals. These stages necessarily include development in knowledge, skills, abilities, and attitudes. By locating the position of a specific course in the curriculum and by comparing its general instructional goals to the goals of the curriculum, the teacher can better determine exactly how the course's content can contribute to the educational needs of students enrolled in the program. Once this view of the course has been established, an examination of the specific learning objectives enables the teacher to define the subject content students should confront to meet these objectives.

The teacher's thinking should also be influenced by the natural or traditional organization of the subject. Some subjects are inherently better organized than others and thus their divisions and boundaries are more clearly recognizable.

The organization or boundaries of a subject include the levels of the subject, i.e., the detailed analyses of individual elements or components, as well as the experimental or research efforts aimed at extending knowledge of the subject. Organization also includes the relationships of the subject to others, whether the relationship is between similar subjects, such as virology and immunology, or between basic-science subjects and clinical applications, such as study of the pancreas and the treatment of diabetes mellitus.

The process of selecting subject content can be illustrated by two sections from two units on the red cell. One unit represents a medical-school hematology course, while the other is designed for a course in hematology in a medical-technology program.

The overall purpose of the medical-school educational program is the preparation of physicians qualified to provide health care at different levels. To this end, a basic-science component provides basic-science principles underlying clinical care through courses in organ systems and systemic diseases. As part of the basic-science program, the hematology course describes the functioning and malfunctioning of the hematologic system. This course therefore contributes to the scientific basis for medical decision making required of medical-school graduates.

The overall purpose of the medical-technology program is the preparation of professional laboratory workers qualified to function in a variety of health-related laboratory environments. To this end, a series of courses emphasizing disease processes and clinical manifestations provides the requisite academic experiences for later professional laboratory work. As part of this series, a hematology course concentrating on the red cell describes red cell development, metabolism, and disease states, as well as specific laboratory procedures. The course therefore contributes to the students' ability to perform procedures and correlate their results with specific diseases or conditions.

A unit on anemia in the medical-school course could concentrate, in part, on the identification and classification of anemias; the morphology and pathologic processes associated with each; their clinical features; the interpretation of corroborating laboratory evidence; the methods of diagnoses employed; and the basic treatment modalities of each.

A unit on anemia in the medical-technology course could concentrate, in part, on the general causes of anemia; the life span of the red cell in normal and anemic states; the types and mechanisms of hemolysis; the performance and interpretation of such procedures as hematocrits, autohemolysis, and incubated quantitative osmotic fragility tests; and the interpretation of peripheral blood smears of patients with selected disease states.

In both units the specific learning objectives are developed in light of the general objectives of both programs. These objectives specify the type of professional to be prepared and indicate the relative position of the hematology courses in their respective curricula. Subject content thus is selected according to specific learning objectives. In the medical-school course, the learning objectives might be directed toward several instructional goals, one of which could be: "Understands the pathophysiologic processes involved in the major anemias." The medical-technology program, on the other hand, could have as one instructional goal: "Evaluates the results of laboratory tests in terms of the characteristics of specific anemias."

Subject content in both units also is selected according to the boundaries of the subject matter of hematology, specifically the red cell and various types of anemias. These boundaries are observed in light of the objectives of both courses. In the medical-school course, for example, students might be introduced to anemia by examining the kinetic classification of anemia in terms of the reticulocyte index. In the medical-technology course students could begin their study of peripheral blood smears by examining the maturation of reticulocytes and then performing reticulocyte counts on peripheral blood.

SEQUENCING SUBJECT CONTENT

The sequencing of subject content is closely associated with the selection of content. Its purpose is to provide an approach to subject content that students will find intellectually satisfactory. The teacher must therefore arrange selected content so that it flows in a continuous, logical, integrated manner.

There is no single correct approach to sequencing content. The process can be affected by several factors. Some of them may be integral to the subject content, such as the sequence of procedures for performing a gingevectomy; others may be extraneous to the course, such as the relative availability of patients, specimens, or materials.

One basic approach to sequencing involves arranging content according to the logical relationships between and among the natural divisions, subdivisions, or boundaries of the subject itself (6). This approach is closely associated with the criteria for selecting content and can include arranging content as it proceeds from the simple to the complex (such as placing the characteristics of specific bacteria before the role of the same bacteria in human disease); from the concrete to the abstract or the known to the experimental (such as placing principles of chemical carcinogenesis before discussions of current chemotherapy research); or according to whole-part or part-whole relationships (such as the series of technical radiographic procedures that contribute to the production of radiographs).

A related approach to sequencing is based on arranging content according to the established manner in which a specific task is performed (6). This approach requires that each of the tasks or skills included in a course be analyzed to identify their component parts and their relationships to other tasks (7). Such an analysis enables a teacher to determine which specific content is needed as prerequisite or corollary to the task. A review of the anatomy and physiology of the thoracic cavity area, for example, would be requisite to learning how to examine the thorax and lungs in a patient-assessment course, while the concepts of consolidation and rale could be approached through simulations and included as part of the demonstrations of examination techniques.

The analysis of tasks also provides the means for determining the sequence of tasks or skills which, when combined, form a complex task students must be able to perform. This sequence should follow as closely as possible the sequence that exists in the laboratory or clinical environment. Thus, the series of content areas and related skills that combine to form a comprehensive patient assessment, for example, should be arranged in the same sequence that students will later be expected to follow as they conduct an assessment.

These approaches to sequencing suggest that students initially be given the opportunity to relate to the subject content scheduled any knowledge or skills they already possess, and that any identified prerequisite knowledge, skills, or attitudes be gained, mastered, or experienced before students advance into more complex areas. They also suggest that, when sequencing content and associated learning experiences, the teacher be aware of any institutional curricular design requirements that may affect sequencing in a particular area, such as established departmental guidelines for the progression of pharmaceutics courses in a pharmacy curriculum. Of further concern should be the time or material resources that could have an effect on how content and activities can be scheduled.

IDENTIFYING RESOURCES AND CONSTRAINTS

When planning to teach, several factors must be considered either individually or in tandem for their potential effects on the way a course can be developed, managed, and evaluated. Depending on the situation, these factors can function as either resources or constraints on a teacher's activities.

One factor involves the *range of abilities and previous knowledge, skills, and experiences that students bring to a particular course.* This range is identified by an assessment of student characteristics conducted at the outset of the course. (Methods for conducting this assessment are discussed in Chapter 4.) Prior to this assessment, new teachers must base their planning on the advice and suggestions of colleagues concerning general student characteristics, while experienced teachers can rely on previous work to guide their initial planning. For both teachers, the results of the assessment provide the basis for finalizing all planning.

Heterogeneous groups of students displaying a variety of backgrounds and preparation levels are found most often in prerequisite or lower-level courses, in elective courses, and even in some clinical rotations. This type of grouping can be a resource if the teacher plans to include discussion sessions, small-group experiences, student instruction of other students, or provisions for individually paced instruction. A heterogeneous grouping can serve as a constraint on planning if the teacher has limited time to spend with students (such as in a two-week in-service course on ostomy care for nurses from different services) or lacks appropriate resources for personalizing instruction (such as being scheduled in a lecture hall with a group of 190 students).

Homogeneous groups of students displaying highly similar backgrounds and preparation levels are found most frequently in advanced courses. Such groups become an obvious resource if the teacher has a limited amount of time to cover extensive subject content. Because of their similar learning styles and ability levels, the students are able to progress readily together through the planned learning experiences. Such groups can be a constraint, however, if the teacher's plans are based on an anticipated diversity of student backgrounds. For example, an interdisciplinary elective course on legal, ethical, and social issues facing the health-care system will necessarily be limited in the perspectives represented if 90 percent of the class is nursing students. Similarly, discussions in a course in human sexuality are bound to suffer if the enrollment is exclusively male.

Another factor that can function as a resource or constraint involves the *amount of time available for a course and its place in the institutional time schedule.* Most elements of the time factor usually are known by teachers in advance of teaching, e.g., length of class period, time of day, duration of the entire course, and the general number of credit hours students usually carry. These elements are usually fixed and most teachers have little or no control over them.

Experienced teachers generally view the time element as a constraint, primarily because traditional lecture-presentation methods must be employed to cover required material or because all students, due to the limited teaching time, must be viewed as possessing similar backgrounds and preparation levels. New teachers may also view the time element as a constraint, because they are inexperienced in selecting content and appropriate teaching methods. Therefore, their planning activities are directed at "covering as much content as possible" in subsequent teaching.

While the time element is a true resource in those infrequent situations where it exists in abundance, as in summer remedial or enrichment programs devoted to a select group of students, it can be also used to the teacher's and students' advantage in more typical situations. This can be accomplished through a combination of activities. One involves using the results of the assessment of student characteristics to identify individual backgrounds, competencies in the subject content, and preferences for methods of learning, so that students can be directed to appropriate learning activities. Closely related activities entail developing a set of alternative teaching-learning methods for use in managing the course, which can range from a detailed reading list, to programmed workbooks, to contingency contracting. While all these activities necessarily require a definite time commitment of the teacher prior to instruction, the efficient use of time they provide in the teaching-learning process more than justifies the effort.

The *relative availability of equipment, materials, and facilities* also acts as a facilitating or limiting factor in planning teaching activities. Access to a media production unit is prerequisite to any considerations of developing videotapes or slide-tape programs to supplement or complement teaching activities. The institutional procedures for scheduling students through clinical rotations necessarily affects not only the selection and sequencing of content, but the manner in which a course is managed; if dialysis patients will be available only after week twelve, it would be futile to sequence renal-failure management at week three.

The potential constraints imposed by a lack of some needed materials can be alleviated somewhat if teachers examine the process involved in developing material resources. Departmental or divisional monies are frequently available for the acquisition or modification of equipment or materials. Teachers beginning their planning activities should investigate the procedures for obtaining and using available funds, such as the requisition process and the typical time lapse from requisition to receipt of ordered material. Teachers should also become familiar with the procedures of the school or department budget committee and the manner in which requests for monies are reviewed by the committee.

In some situations, no money is available for altering or purchasing material and equipment. The potential constraints of such situations can be alleviated if teachers modify their initial plans to include methods or activities that require little or no financial commitment. Simulation exercises, gaming activities, or role playing, among others, are effective teaching-learning methods that entail minimal costs. Such alternatives to limited resources require that teachers familiarize themselves with new procedures or techniques and try them out in the teaching-learning process.

The *financial requirements of methods, materials, and activities* represent potential resources or constraints closely associated with the other factors affecting the planning process. As with the time element, the ready availability of money to develop materials or purchase equipment is an obvious resource, while its typically short supply serves as a constraint on certain activities. Teachers' primary concerns at the beginning of the planning process include determining the previous financial allocations for a course (if it has been taught in the past); the current availability of departmental or division monies for instructional support; and the costs involved in purchasing, developing, or maintaining the materials and equipment to be used in teaching, such as overhead transparencies or tape recorders. The ways in which these concerns are resolved affects not only the planning process, but also later development, management, and evaluation activities.

ALLOCATING INSTRUCTIONAL TIME

The distribution and allocation of instructional time for divisions and sub-divisions of subject content and for specific teaching-learning activities takes place as teachers select and sequence subject content in light of the various resources and constraints they have identified.

There is no one correct way to allocate time in a course. Specific techniques or guidelines for allocating instructional time vary according to the subject-matter requirements of specific courses; teachers' personal competencies in their field; and their previous experience in constructing and managing a course.

Two general approaches can be used to allocate time in most subject-content areas. The first involves *considering the nature of the specific learning objectives of a course.* As teachers develop objectives, they can, at the same time, determine the relative amount of time students will need to achieve them. This includes both the time needed for student-teacher interaction and the time needed for students to work on their own or in groups.

By developing objectives according to the two-level system previously described—i.e., minimal and developmental competence—initial decisions concerning time allocation can be facilitated. Both kinds of objectives implicitly indicate a relative degree of difficulty; they specify whether a particular task is something all students should master, is prerequisite to the performance of other tasks, or is to be developed to the fullest extent possible according to individual abilities. Minimal competence objectives usually require less time of both teachers and students than do developmental competence objectives, which by their nature entail complex activities.

The second approach to allocating time involves *considering student characteristics and the nature of the student-teacher transactions that are to take place.* Knowledge of student characteristics is obtained through the assessment conducted at the outset of a course. Such characteristics as background, prior experience, and pretest results help to identify the collective and individual abilities of the students, their probable readiness to begin work toward various objectives, and the probable rate at which they will be able to proceed.

These characteristics can also be used to guide the final selection of methods and materials. Discovering that students entering a course possess similar characteristics permits the teacher to finalize previous tentative selections, while discovering a diversity in student backgrounds and abilities necessitates incorporating remedial or enrichment self-paced learning activities. In the first instance the homogeneous nature of the students should enable them to proceed through a course at the same pace. A heterogeneous group of students, on the other hand, requires methods and materials geared to differences in students' abilities; these additions necessarily entail more extensive time commitments for student-teacher transactions than were probably planned initially.

SELECTING METHODS AND MATERIALS

Teachers' selections of methods for engaging in transactions with students are initially based on an assessment of their own strengths and weaknesses. Such assessments require that teachers be honest with themselves; if strengths remain unidentified or weaknesses overlooked, the quality of the teaching-learning transactions is adversely affected. Further, the sense of trust teachers must develop with their students can also suffer, for poor discussions or presentations or missed opportunities for alternative methods of teaching can be interpreted by students, sometimes justifiably, as representing a teacher's lack of concern or disinterest in teaching.

Personal strengths in the development and execution of teaching methods can be identified through personal reflection, student evaluations, and peer review or suggestions. Obvious strengths should be used as the foundation for the teaching-learning transaction. Potential strengths, such as those suggested by student or peer evaluations, should be pursued and developed as a teacher becomes more comfortable in teaching and is willing to take the risk of experimenting with something new.

Personal weaknesses in teaching methods can be identified in the same manner as strengths. Once identified and acknowledged by the teacher, two alternatives are usually available. The first involves seeking outside help to revise or refine current methods. This help can be found in such diverse sources as professional or educational journals, experienced colleagues, or a professional, in-service staff-development consultant. If these sources prove unsatisfactory, the second alternative involves discontinuing current methods and trying something new. This is probably more difficult to accomplish than the first, at least initially, but can often be more rewarding. A teacher who has used the lecture-presentation method in a medical-surgical nursing course because other department members lecture, but who feels uncomfortable and unsuccessful doing so, could structure the course around a series of group discussion sessions if personal contact with students poses no threat.

Methods selection is also based on an assessment of students' strengths and weaknesses. Although this assessment takes place at the beginning of a course, its results can serve to solidify initial selections or indicate the need for appropriate alternatives.

Initial methods selections in the planning stage are based on the type of students a teacher has encountered in the past, if previous teaching has been done. Such student characteristics as preferences for learning techniques, entering competencies in the subject content, and previous academic and clinical experience are frequently similar from one course offering to the next. Once the course has begun, specific characteristics of the entering group of students can be identified and the methods selected can be finalized or revised accordingly. If provisions for personalized instruction have been incorporated in past courses for different kinds of students, and the student assessment indicates the new group consists of students of common abilities and interests, then slightly different teaching methods will be needed than were used in the past.

New teachers preparing for the first teaching experience usually have to rely on their colleagues to find out about the characteristics of students they should expect to be teaching. The information they receive through this inquiry process will serve as the basis for initial methods selections; the student assessment carried out at the beginning of their course then assumes added significance for matching methods with students.

Methods selections are also based on the type of learning that is to take place. If the emphasis is to be on factual material, rules, or principles, didactic presentations, ranging from lecture presentations to programmed instruction to independent study, are most appropriate. If student learning of skills is to be emphasized, methods involving maximum student participation (with teacher assistance when necessary) are best. Skills in patient assessment or medical interviewing, for example, could well be taught through use of slide-tape or videotape presentations, role playing, simulations, or small-group work.

Finally, methods selections are also based on programmatic considerations. Each method available to a teacher carries certain time, resource, or institutional requirements. These can include the number of students enrolled in the course; the availability of other instructors, laboratory or teaching assistants, and clerical help; the physical facilities, such as lecture halls or meeting rooms, their location and available space; the number of clinical activities; and the length of class meeting times, content units, or the course as a whole. Each of these factors can be a resource or constraint on both the selection and the execution of teaching methods. Proper planning therefore requires their consideration.

The selection of materials to be used in the teaching-learning process is guided by considerations similar to those for selecting methods. Printed handouts, slide-tapes, programmed-instruction workbooks, or other materials are selected to contribute to students' achievement of objectives; to reflect the strengths of teachers and students, and the type of learning desired; and to capitalize on their respective programmatic requirements.

Materials selections are further guided by the availability of materials already developed for a course, department, or division; by the availability of facilities for developing and producing new materials, such as an illustration/photography department; and by the amount of money available to teachers to purchase materials from other health science units or from commercial publishing houses.

DEVELOPING AN EVALUATION PLAN

A systematic plan for evaluating teaching activities is an integral part of the planning stage. With some understanding of the evaluation process and of what and how they want to evaluate, teachers will find that early planning for evaluation can be accomplished easily and effectively.

Detailed discussions of the evaluation process and specific evaluation activities are presented in Unit 4. These discussions focus on the evaluation of student learning and the effectiveness of the teaching-learning process.

The evaluation of student learning is directed by several basic decisions the teacher must make before any evaluation takes place. Because of the sampling nature of this form of evaluation, initial decisions involve determining which knowledge, skills, abilities, or behaviors are representative of the various objectives and content areas to be covered. The teacher must then decide which devices can best measure these chosen capabilities. Finally, decisions must be made regarding the standards to be used in judging the results of the evaluation process. Standards can be either criterion-referenced, i.e., based on predetermined performance standards representing learning objectives; or norm-referenced, i.e., based on the relative performances of the group of students being evaluated.

Like student learning, the teaching-learning process is a complex, multifaceted phenomenon; to evaluate all its parts in every situation, particularly within the typical constraints of any educational program, would be extremely difficult. The primary aim in evaluating the process, then, is to assess its crucial elements in terms of preestablished criteria. This necessarily implies that both the elements to be evaluated and the criteria to be used are agreed on by all participants in the evaluation process.

The participants in an evaluation of teaching effectiveness can include students, who are asked to provide either verbal or written feedback on an individual or collective basis; the teacher's colleagues, who are asked to assess the development of teaching or to observe parts of the teaching-learning process itself; and the teachers themselves, who can evaluate their own transactions with students through such means as videotaped microteaching.

Teachers committed to providing for the individuality of students attempt to provide alternate pathways for students to work toward course objectives. The material components of these pathways, such as slide-tapes, simulation models, or learning laboratories, must also be evaluated in terms of their relative quality and utility, for they have a direct effect on both the process and the product of teaching-learning transactions. Thus, this evaluation is as significant as the other evaluation activities, and can be conducted by students, teachers, and teachers' colleagues.

In both of these areas, judgments about the relative worth of specific activities cannot be made without reference to valid and reliable data. Developing an evaluation plan as part of the activities of the planning stage allows teachers sufficient time to construct valid and reliable evaluation mechanisms. These mechanisms should be natural extensions of the objectives, content, and materials and resources included in the teaching-learning process.

REFERENCES

1. BIGGE, MORRIS L. *Learning Theories for Teachers.* 2d ed. New York: Harper & Row, 1971.
2. CRONBACH, LEE J. *Essentials of Psychological Testing.* 3d ed. New York: Harper & Row, 1970.
3. GLASER, ROBERT, AND ANTHONY J. NITKO. "Measurement and Learning in Instruction." In Robert L. Thorndike, ed., *Educational Measurement.* 2d ed. Washington, D.C.: American Council on Education, 1970, pp. 625–670.
4. GRONLUND, NORMAN E. *Stating Behavioral Objectives for Classroom Instruction.* New York: Macmillan, 1970.
5. MILLMAN, JASON. "Passing Scores and Test Lengths for Domain-Referenced Measures." *Review of Educational Research* 43 (1973): 205–215.
6. POSNER, GEORGE J., AND KENNETH A. STRIKE. "A Categorization Scheme for Principles of Sequencing Content." *Review of Educational Research* 46 (1976): 665–690.
7. SEGALL, ASCHER J. et al. *Systematic Course Design for the Health Fields.* New York: Wiley, 1975.
8. SMITH, B. OTHANEL, WILLIAM O. STANLEY, AND J. HARLOV SHORES. *Fundamentals of Curriculum Development.* New York: Harcourt, Brace and World, 1957.

4
ASSESSING
STUDENT
CHARACTERISTICS

The ultimate goal of teachers in any health science education program should be systematically to plan teaching and learning activities so that some form of interactive teaching-learning system is achieved. Such a system attempts to be responsive to the needs, interests, and characteristics of individual students. By assessing student characteristics and performance prior to and during the teaching-learning process, the teacher obtains information that makes it possible to adapt the process to each student or group of students. The purpose, of course, is to individualize teaching and learning activities (8).

Individualized teaching and learning, in its ideal form, would have as many different teaching and learning strategies as there are differences in students' methods, rates, and interests in learning. In most health science education programs, even under optimal conditions, individualized teaching and learning is not possible, for it necessitates extensive diagnostic procedures to discover relevant differences in students, followed by the prescription and administration of a multitude of different teaching-learning activities.

While the ideal form of individualized instruction is seldom attainable, certain variations are not only possible but are highly feasible, even for teachers responsible for 100 or more students in an introductory required course. For example, teachers should be able to combine associationist and cognitive approaches to learning to provide opportunities for students to engage in self-directed learning, at least to achieve minimal competence objectives, and then to spend time in groups with the teacher problem solving and working toward developmental competence objectives. The activities available to students to achieve minimal competence objectives could be varied and need not be dependent on the utilization of class time. Thus, where a lecture presentation may have been used to present content and discuss principles, in an interactive teaching-learning system it might be replaced by a series of slide-tape programs or programmed-instruction workbooks. The teacher's decisions in this regard are not whether or not to make different learning opportunities available to students, but rather what kind of opportunities would be most effective and most appropriate for different students. These decisions are best made if information about relevant student characteristics is available.

The assessment of student characteristics is one viable means for teachers to obtain information useful in planning, developing, managing, and evaluating the teaching-learning process. The assessment can be as simple or as complex as resources permit, but, whatever its level of sophistication, such assessment should be an integral part of each teacher's educational activities.

While a variety of student characteristics can be assessed, care should be taken to obtain only information that actually can be used by the teacher and students in their respective decision making. "Information overload" can occur when students and teachers spend a great deal of time at the beginning of a course or unit responding to and analyzing various characteristic inventories. The possibility of generating useless information can be avoided altogether if teachers look on the results of an assessment of student characteristics as a means to further plan and develop a course or unit, as well as to manage and evaluate it. The results can also be a means for guiding students and providing direction through a course or unit. Only information that relates to the way the course is conducted should therefore be collected. Information not immediately usable can be collected to guide later planning and development activities, e.g., the selection and development of various types of media resources.

Any assessment of student characteristics should be conducted at the beginning of the course or unit. This will serve to assist students in self-assessment, prepare them for the course and the alternative activities and resources it provides, and indicate the teacher's interest in them as individuals.

APPROACHES TO ASSESSING STUDENT CHARACTERISTICS

Teachers committed to the concept that students can be responsible for their own learning if given the opportunity will want to increase the number of opportunities for student self-directed learning. To be valid and ultimately effective, such opportunities should be developed on the basis of information about relevant student characteristics. "Relevant" here refers to characteristics associated with a student's approach to learning.

Some students prefer to be totally self-directed in their learning, while others require the constant attention and direction of a teacher. Some are fact oriented and have little difficulty in recalling information, while others are concept oriented and have little difficulty in problem solving. In addition, each of these types of students may or may not possess skills in reading and reading comprehension or in studying, note taking, or test taking, factors that affect their general learning approaches. Any of these elements can have a bearing on the type of learning activity that would be most effective and therefore most appropriate for different types of students. The teacher must therefore determine which approaches or factors are most common in the students being taught, which ones have the greatest potential impact on the overall teaching-learning process, and which ones can be dealt with effectively and efficiently during the development process.

Several types of relevant student characteristics can be assessed, depending on teachers' purposes in teaching and the resources they have at their disposal. Teachers assessing student characteristics for the first time should use the results they obtain to guide the subsequent planning and development of alternative teaching-learning activities. Later assessments, conducted after some teaching experience has been achieved, can be used to counsel students in their selection of appropriate learning activities.

Factors that Affect Students' Approaches to Learning

A variety of factors can have a positive or negative effect on students' approaches to learning. Such factors as reading ability, note-taking skills, or study methods can play an important role in the degree of success realized, regardless of the specific educational program in which a student is enrolled. These factors often go unnoticed by teachers, however, who misinterpret their effects and incorrectly attribute them to students' disinterest in subject content, lack of motivation, or some similar disability.

In an ideal situation, a study-skills counselor or reading specialist would have faculty status in an educational program and be charged with developing and conducting programwide self-improvement opportunities for students. These specialists would also be available to individual faculty members to assist them and their students in developing appropriate skills within the context of a specific course or unit of study.

The ideal situation and such specialists are unfortunately few in number. At best, most health science schools, departments, and faculty members rely on the services provided by a central group of specialists serving an entire campus or institution, e.g., a Dean of Students Office. Frequently, reading and study-skills assistance must come from some outside source, such as a vocational-technical school or local school district. If services, in whatever form, are available, so that difficulties experienced by students can be followed up and treated, teachers should be encouraged to develop at least an awareness of the common manifestations of the difficulties so that they may suggest remedial work when appropriate.

Unlike other forms of student-characteristic assessment, the determination of student deficiencies in reading or study skills can be done on an informal, individual basis. Instead of conducting formal diagnostic testing sessions with all students at the beginning of a course or unit, an activity outside the professional purview of most health science teachers, the teacher should be prepared to identify those weaknesses or deficiencies that will have an effect on student performance. Reading skills, for example, while essential for students in any course, are requisite to success in introductory courses covering extensive amounts of factual material. Just as good readers would be expected to be more familiar with words and their usage, have a better vocabulary, and be able to read faster and comprehend what they read, the poor readers lacking these skills are likely to experience difficulty in assimilating, comprehending, and later recalling information obtained from written sources (11). Similarly, study, memory, and concentration skills are also essential for student success. Students with well-developed skills will be more likely to participate successfully in various teaching-learning activities, while students deficient in these skills may sit through lectures without taking notes, fail to finish examinations or assignments, or require inordinate amounts of time to accomplish what others can do easily and efficiently (5).

If teachers can anticipate problems caused by student weaknesses in reading or study skills and develop the ability to assess such weaknesses through observation, misinterpretation of student learning difficulties can be avoided and the students can be referred to specialists for remedial help.

Learning Style

One student characteristic that teachers can assess as part of their planning and development activities is the learning style of their students. Learning style refers to a student's orientation to or preference for techniques for learning; it indicates the general manner in which a particular student prefers to engage in the teaching-learning process.

Assessments of learning styles have been developed and conducted in some institutions and used on both schoolwide and departmental bases. Although developed locally, and therefore reflections of the educational goals or philosophies of specific schools or departments, learning-style or learning-preference inventories have generally attempted to assess similar characteristics. The most common characteristics assessed have been student preferences for self-directed or other-directed learning (4,9). A preference for self-directed or independent learning indicates students' interest in learning approaches that are relatively unstructured and informal, approaches that allow them to set their own goals and pursue their own interests. A preference for other-directed learning activities indicates students' needs for structured, formal teaching-learning activities with specific, clear-cut guidelines, direction, and evaluation. The assessment of these two general orientations to learning has also been combined with assessments of other cognitive and affective factors, so that a student's learning preference can also indicate the degree to which such things as abstract or concrete content and working alone or with others are preferred techniques or methods of learning (7).

Students' learning styles are usually assessed by asking students to respond to a series of questions or statements describing specific learning techniques, e.g., "I would rather work with others on a project than work on it by myself," or, "Audiovisual materials are more helpful than written resources provided by the teacher." Students respond to each question or statement by using a multipoint, Likert-type response scale to indicate the extent of their agreement or disagreement. On a seven-point scale, for example, 1 might represent strong agreement with the statement, while 7 might represent strong disagreement. The total responses of each student are then analyzed using a conversion scale, factor analysis, or some similar technique to obtain a numerical style or preference score.

Teachers can develop their own learning-style assessment devices for use with students in their courses. The assessment device can be as simple or as complex as the teacher's purposes and resources warrant. At the very least, it should contain questions or statements reflecting the activities and resources that will be available in the course. Students can respond to each with a simple "yes" or "no" or "agree" or "disagree." A tally of their responses should then provide a general description of their orientation to or preference for learning techniques.

The information from a teacher's assessment of students' learning styles would be particularly useful, for example, if alternative teaching-learning activities have been developed and are available; if students can choose between attending in-class sessions or working on their own; or if different resources dealing with the same objectives are available for student use. The information could be used at the outset of a course or unit to assist students in examining their own approaches to learning and in selecting appropriate learning activities. It could also be used at the end of a course or unit for evaluation purposes, either in evaluating specific learning activities or resources or in evaluating the overall effectiveness of the course.

Cognitive Preference Style

The assessment of a second student characteristic, cognitive preference style, can become another area of potentially fruitful investigation for teachers interested in developing an interactive teaching-learning system. Cognitive preference style refers to a student's preferred method of approaching and dealing with content. It may be stable across different subjects, or it may change from one subject area to another. For example, a student may prefer to deal with biological information in terms of the basic priniciples underlying it, but at the same time deal with sociological information on a recall basis only. Because it is related to students' approaches to specific subject content, cognitive preference style can be used by teachers to guide students to one of several strategies available for learning specific content, or to reinforce or redirect students' approaches to the subject content of a particular course.

Cognitive preference style usually refers to students' preferences for one of our different modes or approaches to scientific information (10);

- *Recall:* the acceptance of information for its own sake, i.e., without consideration of its implications, applications, or limitations.
- *Principles:* the acceptance of information because it exemplifies or explains some fundamental scientific principle or relationship.
- *Questioning:* the critical questioning of information as regards its completeness, general validity, or limitations.
- *Application:* the acceptance of information in view of its usefulness and applicability in a general, social, or scientific context.*

Measures of cognitive preference style are obtained by developing and administering a multiple-choice test dealing with specific subject content. The test is comprised of items that have four options; each option is a correct answer to the question or statement contained in the item. Students mark the option they feel is most intellectually satisfying. By summarizing the student's responses to all items of the test, a response pattern becomes apparent, permitting the identification of a cognitive preference style. A student selecting a greater percentage of recall-referenced options, for example, would indicate an overall preference for a recall mode of approaching subject content.

Teachers can develop their own subject-content tests to determine students' cognitive preference styles. Similar tests, already developed and administered in various situations, have usually consisted of 20 to 30 items. Because students must be familiar with subject content to make a valid preference choice (1), the items developed should refer to content students have already encountered and that is related to the content of the course they are beginning.

The following test item, taken from one of the first assessment devices developed to determine cognitive preference style (2), illustrates the general approach to item construction:

The pressure of a gas is directly proportional to its absolute temperature.

(Questioning) A. The statement, as given, fails to consider effects of volume changes and change of state.

(Recall)   B. Charles's or Gay-Lussac's Law.

(Principles)   C. The statement implies a lower limit to temperature.

---

*From P. Tamir, "The Relationship among Cognitive Preference, School Environment, Teachers' Curricular Bias, Curriculum, and Subject Matter," *American Educational Research Journal,* Summer 1975, p. 236. Copyright © 1975, American Educational Research Association, Washington, D.C.

(Application) D.   This principle is related to the fact that overheated automobile tires may "blow out."*

The designations to the left of the options above (excluded on the test itself) indicate the general manner in which options are developed to refer to one of the four modes or approaches to information. They also indicate how test results are used. Students selecting option A in the example would be adding to their "Questioning" preference measure; selection of option B would add to their "Recall" preference measure; and so on. While students will not consistently choose one type of option as the answer to all questions, the final pattern of their responses will emphasize one preference mode over the other three.

The assessment of cognitive preference style often provides useful information for educational decisions teachers and students make during the progress of a course or unit. While this type of assessment is especially appropriate for use by individual teachers, it may also prove highly effective when used on a departmental or divisional level. Individual results could be used for counseling students and managing individual courses; group results could be used in evaluating the process and the product of the overall educational program.

Cognitive Style

A third type of student characteristic, cognitive style, represents the manner in which students perform cognitive tasks. Cognitive style refers to an individual's typical modes of perceiving, remembering, thinking, and problem solving (3). It is the characteristic approach or "style" individuals bring to a wide range of situations. Because this approach encompasses both perceptual and intellectual activities, it is termed their "cognitive" style.

Cognitive style differs from the cognitive preference style just discussed in that the former is measured through use of a variety of psychological tests or test batteries requiring sophisticated analysis and interpretation techniques. In this respect it is beyond the scope and resources of most teachers, for a thorough understanding of the psychological theories, constructs, and techniques underlying it are requisite to its use. Further, while extensive, basic research has been conducted on cognitive style over the last twenty years, much remains to be done on its practical applications and implications for higher education in general and health science education in particular. Despite these reservations, cognitive style merits discussion here because of the potential it holds for planning, developing, managing, and evaluating teaching-learning activities. Teachers should, there-

---

*From R.W. Heath, "Curriculum, Cognition, and Educational Measurement," *Educational and Psychological Measurement* 24 (1964): 243. Reprinted by permission.

fore, become acquainted with the concept of cognitive style, be aware of the contributions its study has already made to education, and anticipate the potential applications that further research may reveal.

Several dimensions of cognitive style have already been identified, among them the individual's manner of processing information, dealing with distractions or cognitive interference, tolerating ambiguity, and forming concepts (3). These dimensions are based on bipolar attributes, so that an individual will be described as possessing one or the other attribute of a particular dimension. The most extensively researched dimension has been "field independence-field dependence"; this dimension refers to an individual's tendency to perceive things in either an analytical or a global fashion. An individual described as field independent, or analytic, experiences things apart from their backgrounds, deals with things outside the context in which they are found. The person who tends to be field dependent or global in approach, however, perceives the overall picture; his or her perception of an item is dominated by the organization of the background or context in which that item is found (13).

Data from research conducted on the field independence-field dependence dimension illustrate its potential applications to educational situations. Individuals who are relatively field dependent have been found to experience difficulty with problems whose solutions depend on taking some critical element out of the context in which it is presented and restructuring the problem material (12). A field-dependent student, for example, may be successful in learning the elements and sequence of the physical diagnosis in a didactic-oriented course, but unsuccessful in using the diagnosis format when dealing with actual patients in a clinical setting.

Field-dependent individuals have also been found to experience more difficulty than field-independent individuals in learning material that lacks some inherent structure and that requires them to provide whatever organization is needed for learning (12). Field-independent students would therefore be more likely to be successful in an independent study environment, where they are given a list of learning objectives, resources, and materials and independently determine their own learning approach and rate of progress.

Analytic or field-independent individuals generally perform well on structured tasks requiring the abstraction of relevant material, while global or field-dependent individuals show more processing of social cues and greater social sensitivity. In this regard, field-independent nurses were found to perform better in surgical nursing, while moderately field-dependent nurses were found to perform better in psychiatric nursing (6). While further study is needed, cognitive style may be useful in career counseling to help ensure a degree of "fit" between students' perceptual and intellectual orientations and the specific professional area of concentration they choose.

REFERENCES

1. ATWOOD, RONALD K. "Development of Cognitive Preference Examination Using General Science and Social Science Content." *Journal of Research in Science Teaching* 8 (1971): 273–275.

2. HEATH, ROBERT W. "Curriculum, Cognition, and Educational Measurement." *Educational and Psychological Measurement* 24 (1964): 239–253.

3. MESSICK, SAMUEL. "The Criterion Problem in the Evaluation of Instruction: Assessing Possible, Not Just Intended, Outcomes." In M. C. Wittrock and David E. Wiley, eds., *The Evaluation of Instruction*. New York: Holt, Rinehart and Winston, 1970, pp. 183–202.

4. MORSTAIN, BARRY R. "Changes in Students' Educational Attitudes: A Study of an Experimental Living-Learning Program." *Research in Higher Education* 1 (1973): 141–148.

5. PAUK, WALTER. *How to Study in College.* 2d ed. Boston: Houghton Mifflin, 1974.

6. QUINLIN, DONALD M., AND SIDNEY J. BLATT. "Field Articulation and Performance Under Stress: Differential Predictions in Surgical and Psychiatric Nursing Training." *Journal of Consulting and Clinical Psychology* 39 (1972): 517.

7. REZLER, AGNES G., AND RUTH M. FRENCH. "Personality Types and Learning Preferences of Students in Six Allied Health Professions." *Journal of Allied Health* 4 (1975): 20–26.

8. STOLUROW, LAWRENCE M. "Summary and Perspectives." In Lawrence M. Stolurow, Theodore I. Peterson, and Anne M. Cunningham, eds., *Computer Assisted Instruction in the Health Professions*. Newburyport, Mass.: Entelek, 1970, pp. 241–258.

9. STONE, HOWARD L., AND HARRY J. KNOPKE. *The Development and Implementation of an Evaluation Model for an Experiment in Planned Curricular Change,* Madison: The University of Wisconsin Center for Health Sciences, 1976.

10. TAMIR, P. "The Relationship Among Cognitive Preference, School Environment, Teacher's Curricular Bias, Curriculum, and Subject Matter." *American Educational Research Journal* 12 (Summer 1975): 235–264.

11. TODD, WILLIAM B., AND CLEMM C. KESSLER. "Influence of Response Mode, Sex, Reading Ability, and Level of Difficulty of Four Measures of Recall of Meaningful Written Material." *Journal of Educational Psychology* 62 (1971): 229–234.

12. WITKIN, H. A. et al. "Field-Dependent and Field-Independent Cognitive Styles and Their Educational Implications." *Review of Educational Research* 47 (1977): 1–64.

13. WITKIN, H. A. et al. *Psychological Differentiation.* New York: Wiley, 1962.

UNIT 1
BIBLIOGRAPHY

Approaches to the Teaching-Learning Process

BAYLES, ERNEST E. *The Theory and Practice of Teaching*. New York: Harper & Row, 1950.

A standard work, presenting a comprehensive view of teaching and learning based on the goal-insight theory. Can be used as a basic reference for study of the cognitive approach to the teaching-learning process.

BIGGE, MORRIS L. *Learning Theories for Teachers*. 3d ed. New York: Harper & Row, 1976.

Presents a clear, lucid discussion of the major approaches to teaching and learning. Compares and contrasts the elements of the associationist and cognitive approaches, describing the implications of each for teachers and for students.

BRUNER, JEROME S. *The Process of Education*. Cambridge, Mass.: Harvard University Press, 1960.

A short, readable report of a conference of scientists and educators dealing with the improvement of science education in primary and secondary schools. The basic principles associated with the conclusions of the conference, that teaching should emphasize the structure of subject content rather than mastery of facts, are applicable to all levels of science education.

GAGNE, ROBERT M. *The Conditions of Learning*. 2d ed. New York: Holt, Rinehart and Winston, 1970.

An associationist approach to teaching and learning. Discusses the conditions for learning associated with eight classes of behavior or performance change.

HILGARD, ERNEST R., and GORDON H. BOWER. *Theories of Learning*. 3d ed. New York: Appleton-Century-Crofts, 1966.

A systematic, detailed discussion of the major psychological theories of learning. Compares and contrasts associationist and cognitive approaches in a clear, readable manner.

SHULMAN, LEE S., and EVAN R. KEISLER, eds. *Learning by Discovery: A Critical Appraisal.* Chicago: Rand McNally, 1966.

A series of papers and dialogues presented by prominent educators and psychologists. Although an older book, it provides one of the better comprehensive treatments of the learning by discovery approach, covering a variety of issues, from research results to practical applications to psychological and educational implications.

SKINNER, B. F. *The Technology of Teaching.* New York: Appleton-Century-Crofts, 1968.

Applies principles of contingency reinforcement to classroom situations. Discusses his associationist approach to teaching and learning in more practical terms than some of his other books or essays.

Planning to Teach

BLOCK, JAMES H., ed. *Mastery Learning.* New York: Holt, Rinehart and Winston, 1971.

Presents several papers dealing with a variety of issues, strategies, and procedures associated with mastery learning. Combines theory, research, and practice considerations. Useful as a basic reference and as an aid for developing teaching-learning units directed at minimal competence objectives.

GAGNE, ROBERT M., and LESLIE J. BRIGGS. *Principles of Instructional Design.* New York: Holt, Rinehart and Winston, 1974.

An associationist-oriented, systematic approach to designing teaching-learning activities. Discusses principles of selecting teaching-learning strategies appropriate to several classifications of learning objectives.

GRONLUND, NORMAN E. *Stating Behavioral Objectives for Classroom Instruction.* New York: Macmillan, 1970.

A concise, straightforward, practical guide to preparing objectives for teaching and testing. Provides specific guidelines for writing instructional goals and specific learning objectives. Appendices include a checklist for evaluating the adequacy of newly written objectives and lists of illustrative verbs that can be used in writing objectives directed at a variety of learning outcomes.

MILLER, HARRY B. *Teaching and Learning in Adult Education.* New York: Macmillan, 1964.

Describes teaching-learning principles and practices appropriate to the adult learner. While concerned with the general area of adult education, many of the book's techniques and strategies should be highly useful for teachers in the health services.

POSNER, GEORGE J., and KENNETH A. STRIKE. "A Categorization Scheme for Principles of Sequencing Content." *Review of Educational Research* 46 (Fall 1976): 665–690.

Discusses principles underlying five approaches to sequencing subject content; the approaches are based on five categories of content elements and their structural relationships. Highly useful reference for systematic planning of teaching-learning activities.

SEGALL, ASCHER J. et al. *Systematic Course Design for the Health Fields.* New York: Wiley, 1975.

Presents an overview approach to designing a course. Its major contribution to teachers planning a course is its comprehensive treatment of the development and use of task analyses, i.e., information concerning actual professional performance and expected student performance. Discusses in cursory fashion specific teaching-learning techniques and strategies.

Assessing Student Characteristics

GAGNE, ROBERT M., ed. *Learning and Individual Differences.* Columbus, Ohio: Merrill, 1967.

A collection of papers dealing with ways individuals differ in their learning and approaches to measuring these individual differences. Discussions include implications for and applications to the teaching-learning process at various levels.

WEISGERBER, ROBERT A., ed. *Perspectives in Individualized Learning.* Itasca, Ill.: Peacock, 1971.

A collection of theory- and practice-oriented papers discussing various approaches to individual differences. Describes the measurement and accommodation of individual differences, and their implications for developing teaching-learning activities. Many papers are oriented to primary- and secondary-level education, but the principles they propose are generally applicable across levels.

WITKIN, H. A. et al. "Field-Dependent and Field-Independent Cognitive Styles and Their Educational Implications." *Review of Educational Research* 47 (1977): 1–64.

A comprehensive analysis of the research involving cognitive styles conducted over the last several decades. Emphasizes research of field-dependence and field-independence. Discusses implications of research results for educational practice.

WITKIN, H. A. et al. *Psychological Differentiation.* New York: Wiley, 1962.

A relatively clear explication of the foundations of cognitive style. An early work, but still used as a basis for much of the research and practical applications of cognitive style.

UNIT 2
THE
DEVELOPMENT
PROCESS

The teaching-learning process evolves through the combination of several different elements: the characteristics of the teacher and students, the nature of learning objectives and subject content, and the composition and sequence of specific learning activities. To accommodate and coordinate these elements to ensure later successful learning requires a systematic approach to planning and development activities.

The planning process establishes the teaching-learning framework. It is within this framework that students will later develop and express themselves as individual learners, accepting responsibility for their own learning. The development process formalizes strategies and materials comprising the proposed framework for use in managing transactions with students. It results in the initial substantive elements of the teaching-learning process, providing a bridge between the plans for teaching and actual teaching-learning transactions.

The overall purpose of the development process is to create opportunities for students to be flexible in their approaches to learning by providing a variety of teaching-learning activities. To arrange for this variety so that students may later pursue specific objectives according to their individual preferences for learning requires a significant commitment of time and effort. This commitment may or may not be recognized by the institutional reward system; it will, however, be rewarded by student performance in the teaching-learning process.

The chapters of this unit provide an overview of the activities of the development process. Chapter 5 deals with the production of media to be employed as teaching-learning strategies. It discusses a variety of media forms teachers can develop themselves. In Chapter 6, simulation games are described as an approach that, although frequently appropriate, is often overlooked by teachers as they develop their courses. Course syllabi and learning packages are discussed in Chapter 7. They represent the skeletal framework around which the activities of the teaching-learning process are organized.

5
INSTRUCTIONAL
MEDIA

Different types of material resources are available to teachers to facilitate the activities they plan to include in the teaching-learning process. Traditional resources, such as textbooks, journals, models, and clinical or laboratory equipment, can make important contributions, as can an array of media resources, such as films, slide-tape programs, tape recordings, and computerized materials.

Instructional media can serve many purposes and can be used in a variety of ways. One or another form of media can provide an alternative to printed materials, a vehicle for displaying specific content or skills, a means for student self-analysis, or even a structured learning experience. Media can be used in class with large groups of students, by a small group of students working together, or by individual students studying independently. The purposes and uses of media are limited only by a teacher's course requirements, resources, personal aptitude for teaching, and imagination.

To teachers who have had minimal experience with instructional media, an introduction to the variety of media resources available for use can be overwhelming or overstimulating. It can be overwhelming if teachers feel incapable of selecting one or two needed resources from the myriad interesting resources confronting them; it can be overstimulating if teachers take a carte-blanche approach and order as much media as they and the budget can tolerate. Both extremes can be avoided if a systematic approach is taken to selecting and using instructional media in a course or unit.

Because instructional media serve to complement or supplement the activities comprising the teaching-learning process, a media resource should be chosen in terms of how it relates to the learning objectives directing particular activities. Thus, the development of media begins with the question, "Which objectives are to be achieved, and how can they best be achieved?'' followed by, ''Which instructional media resources might best help students achieve these objectives?'' Like any other teaching activity, systematic planning for media is necessary before development, management, and evaluation can take place.

PLANNING FOR INSTRUCTIONAL MEDIA

In developing an instructional medium for a course or unit, teachers first complete related planning activities to ensure that quality instructional media resources are sought out or produced. Planning activities are too frequently seen as unnecessary or too time consuming, and teachers, departments, or schools may be tempted to leap ahead and undertake significant instructional media development without the foundation proper planning provides.

When planning to incorporate media resources in a course, teachers first *decide exactly where in the course instructional media are to be used.* While this may seem an obvious and simple task, time, money, and material resources can easily be misspent if only general ideas guide the development process.

Identifying these areas will be easier for the experienced teacher than for new teachers. Experienced teachers can draw on a knowledge of how subject content has been treated in the past; on a familiarity with students' learning styles and their preferences for various learning techniques; and on an understanding of the relative effectiveness of their own contributions to the teaching-learning process. These personal resources are not available to new teachers, and probably will not be available until a course has been taught at least once, or more likely several times. The most reasonable approach available to new teachers may therefore be to become familiar with the types and uses of instructional media resources, so that these resources can be considered for future use while the first teaching experience unfolds.

When a specific content area has been identified as appropriate for media use, its *corresponding learning objectives are assessed in terms of their levels or functions.* Here teachers distinguish between objectives that entail fundamental activities, such as defining, describing, identifying, or selecting, and objectives that entail more complex activities, such as analyzing, performing, interpreting, or demonstrating.

Minimal competence objectives that involve fundamental approaches to specific content and that are prerequisite to later objectives involving problem solving or decision making can usually be achieved through such ''motionless'' media as slide-tapes or programmed instruction (6). A review of statistical concepts and computation methods for an introductory applied research methods course, for example, can be accomplished by students proceeding through a programmed workbook. This media form would be appropriate to the specific objectives and content under consideration, for it effectively provides the means for students to confront and master basic content.

Developmental competence objectives that involve complex content can usually be approached through media that involve motion and provide an opportunity to observe, interpret, or analyze specific skills, situations, or patient behaviors (6). A videotape of the neurological examination will not only demonstrate the components of the examination, it will assist students later in conducting the examination themselves. This form of media would be appropriate to the specific objectives and content being considered, for it provides the means for students to observe the performance and listen to explanations of specific examination procedures, and then proceed with their own problem-solving activities associated with the examination.

Teachers can also *consider the results of the assessment of student characteristics* when planning for media resources. The assessment conducted at the beginning of the teaching-learning process can provide such information as the students' learning styles, their preferences for various teaching and learning techniques, and their individual strengths and weaknesses.

A knowledge of student characteristics can assist the teacher's decisions regarding both the selection and use of particular media resources. Students with reading problems would be more likely to achieve specific objectives by using a slide-tape program than they would by working through a programmed text. Lower-ability students may benefit more than those of higher ability from active participation and response during an instructional-materials presentation; a programmed-instruction unit would be more appropriate for these students (2).

Just as a knowledge of student characteristics can contribute significantly to this planning process, so too can a teacher's knowledge of personal strengths and weaknesses. Teachers using media for the first time will be successful in the long run if their commitment to the use of media is communicated to their students and if they have the patience needed for media to be accepted by the students.

During the planning process teachers begin to *investigate the availability of financial and material resources* that will eventually be required for developing media units. Is there a budget for media, or are there funds that can be applied to media development? Are material resources presently available, such as media already owned or studio facilities and technician time? The status of such resources will have a direct effect on the nature and scope of media development teachers will be able to undertake.

Finally, as plans for specific media near completion, *decisions must be made about the evaluation that will accompany the resource.* Evaluation of the quality and effectiveness of the media resource should grow directly out of the specific learning objectives it is intended to help students achieve. This evaluation can be conducted on completion of the media experience. Students might be asked, for example, to respond to a posttest dealing with content and a questionnaire dealing with the quality of the resource. Evaluation can also be conducted as part of the media experience itself, as when students are asked to react immediately to procedures purposely conducted incorrectly or incompletely, or to respond to a checklist form while a procedure is in progress.

GENERAL APPROACHES TO SELECTING INSTRUCTIONAL MEDIA

Teachers beginning the development of instructional media resources often are disappointed to find that little research evidence exists to help them choose the most effective medium for their own teaching purposes and situations (3). Despite the abundance of research on instructional media conducted at all educational levels, only a relatively few studies have directly examined the instructional effectiveness of different media forms. As a result, decisions to purchase or develop media resources have been based primarily on administrative and organization requirements or considerations, such as cost, availability, and user preference (5).

One general approach to selecting instructional media that acknowledges existing effectiveness evidence and provides latitude for administrative considerations stipulates that, for purely instructional purposes, the selection of media is contingent on the teaching-learning strategies to be employed for particular objectives (8). This approach identifies types of media according to their relationship to the conditions for learning presaging a particular teaching strategy; media forms are therefore classified as either "active carriers" or "passive carriers" of learning conditions.

An active carrier imposes particular conditions of learning on the way subject content is presented through a medium—for example, it may require the delivery of feedback to students at preselected intervals. Such a media resource would be selected for specific objectives to provide students with the amount of practice appropriate to the complexity of the content or skill to be learned. It might also be selected to provide feedback to students based on their ability or on the nature of their performance. Media resources functioning as active carriers of conditions for learning include the various types of programmed instruction and computer-assisted instruction.

A passive carrier does not in itself impose special conditions necessary for learning. It is neutral to the requirements of particular learning conditions and may accommodate different sets of requirements in the same or different teaching-learning situations. The material that is presented or the way it is presented may suggest learning conditions, but the medium itself does not. For example, the repetition of the spelling and pronunciation of prefixes, suffixes, and root words throughout an introductory medical-terminology unit represents a learning condition, but the audiotape presenting the unit does not.

Media resources considered to be passive carriers of conditions for learning include films, television-videotapes, slide-tapes, and audiotapes.

Media resources functioning as active or passive carriers of learning conditions can assist students in different ways in achieving or approaching specific learning objectives. The selection of an active carrier indicates that both the content and the form of a presentation will specify how learning takes place. The selection of a passive carrier indicates that only content will direct learning; the medium presenting it is chosen for other reasons, such as teacher preference or availability of production resources.

Specific characteristics associated with different media forms also influence the manner in which a media resource assists students in attaining objectives. These characteristics need to be considered in any selection decision.

A second general approach to selecting instructional media that complements the first is based on considering media forms in terms of visuals, color, motion, and flexibility (9). *Visuals* may or may not be important for achieving specific objectives, and therefore may or may not be required of a media resource. Students should be able to see the procedures involved in a physical examination of the cardiovascular system if they are to be able to conduct an examination themselves. Thus, a videotape may be an appropriate choice for this section of a physical-diagnosis course. On the other hand, students need only hear examples of the various sounds to be able to differentiate normal and abnormal heart sounds.

Color can sometimes be an important characteristic to consider in the development of visual-containing media. Color visuals are as commonly available as black-and-white; further, the addition of color enhances the overall effect of almost any presentation. Sometimes, however, color can add significantly to purchase or production costs; this can be an unnecessary addition when color is not essential for specific objectives.

An objective involving the identification and interpretation of changes in the optic fundus, for example, requires that Kodachrome slides be produced for a slide-tape program associated with the objective. An objective related to the interpretation of data charts and graphs, however, would not require color visuals. If overhead transparencies had been the media selected here, black-on-white transparencies would be appropriate, as well as less expensive to make than color transparencies.

Motion is oftentimes a requirement of media resources developed for specific objectives. Motion would be essential, for example, for demonstrating the physiologic functions of the carotid sinus and aortic nerve; a film or videotape would be most appropriate in this instance. Procedures or processes involving action may also be displayed through some motionless media, such as a slide-tape, if learning objectives relate to specific steps comprising the procedure or process. While the components of the mental-status examination can be identified and described through stop-action sequences in a videotaped patient interview, they could also be effectively shown through use of the slide-tape format.

Flexibility refers to the degree to which students can use a media resource in different locations or at different times. In general, a media resource is flexible if students can use it anywhere at any time; it is either less flexible or inflexible if student use is restricted by time or equipment considerations. Flexibility can be a highly variable characteristic, depending on the requirements and resources of a department or school. In one situation, for example, students' use of computer-assisted instructional programs may be very flexible: they may be allowed to use the programs themselves in a variety of locations at a variety of times, even at home on portable terminals. In another situation, student use of similar programs may be restricted to certain hours in a learning resource center when computer time is available.

These general approaches to selecting instructional media can serve as initial guidelines for developing the medium most appropriate for specific learning objectives. By extension, they can also contribute a great deal to avoiding later problems of overutilization or underutilization (8) that teachers sometimes face. Underutilization of a media resource occurs when the medium selected has capabilities not required and not used for a particular objective, e.g., a videotape used to display motionless, static material. Overutilization occurs when the selected medium lacks display or response capabilities necessary for certain objectives, e.g., an attempt to simulate the action of the stages of labor and delivery with a slide-tape program. Either condition can occur when the medium is not entirely appropriate to the specific learning objectives. An understanding of the nature of certain objectives and the general characteristics of different instructional media forms, combined with a willingness to engage in systematic media resource development, in almost all instances precludes later problems of utilization.

DEVELOPING MEDIA RESOURCES

Once a specific media form has been selected for use in a course or unit, its development begins with a *review of materials that are currently available for purchase.* Since most teachers' educational expertise centers on their direct involvement with students, not with the production of media, they will frequently find it is more efficient to purchase professional, commercial products than to make their own.

A teacher's review will be aided greatly by consulting a resource person knowledgeable about commercial media. These individuals can be found in the college or university library, in the department providing educational services for health science faculty and staff, or in the instructional-materials center of particular schools or departments. Additional resources to assist the review include the *National Medical Audiovisual Center Catalogue* (13), and the *Index to Health and Safety Education (Multimedia)* (12), which contain most new offerings in the health sciences. The promotional materials for media sent to deans, directors, or department chairmen and the media articles and advertisements contained in professional journals are also sources of information.

If the review process is successful and one or more media resources appear to meet initial selection criteria, a preview of materials should precede purchase. Although this activity is essential for avoiding inappropriate or unusable material, it is becoming increasingly difficult to carry out. Many companies no longer permit previewing, since in the past their materials have been duplicated while out on preview. Some, however, still allow previewing on receipt of a preview charge or the full price of the media, often with the option of a refund if the material is returned.

Under existing circumstances, the process of obtaining sufficient information about materials to be purchased is time consuming and teachers may be tempted to instead produce their own. The situation is admittedly an unsatisfactory one. Many teachers, schools, and departments have devoted time, money, and energy to making media productions that are repetitive and inferior to professional materials they could have purchased. It is therefore essential that time be allotted for investigating currently available media. Only the teacher can formulate a final judgment as a result of actually previewing the material, of course, but much of the searching and administrative work can be done by students, secretaries, or librarians. Teachers should get as much help as they can.

A preview of any commercially produced media resource is conducted primarily to determine whether the resource is suitable for the course's learning objectives and the intended audience. The following general questions (4) can be useful in assessing other important characteristics in the preview process as well as in the selection of most forms of commercially produced media:

1. Is the *content* of the resource significant, accurate, up-to-date? Is it presented at an appropriate level of difficulty and sophistication for the students who will be using the resource?

2. Is the medium *appropriate* to the content? Are requisite characteristics provided for by the medium, e.g. motion, sound, visuals?

3. Is the *cost* of the resource in line with the educational results likely to be obtained by its use? Would another, less expensive resource, perhaps another media form, be a better choice? Or should more money be allocated to acquire a more complex or sophisticated resource?

4. Is the *technical quality* satisfactory? Are photography, illustrations, layout, editing, typeface, and sound appealing or distracting, adequate or inadequate? (Some professional assistance may be needed here.)

5. Is the resource likely to function effectively in the *intended circumstances of use*? Will it be suitable for large groups, small groups, independent study, in-class presentations, or at-home study?

6. Is *validation evidence* supplied by the publisher? Are data available that detail the development of the resource through systematic trial and revision? Has the resource been studied in experimental situations with groups of students similar to those for whom the resource is intended?*

Once the preview process has been completed, distinctions have been made between what can be purchased and what must be developed and produced locally, and the decision has been made to develop a particular media resource, the specifics of each media form need to be considered in terms of *purpose, budget,* and *production*.

Videotape

Videotape is a complex, sophisticated media form. The pieces of equipment needed to use videotape are more elaborate than those used for other forms. It also requires more equipment and technological expertise to produce, and production costs can be very high.

The obvious medium to contrast it with is film. Videotape's major disadvantage is that it is not precisely photographic—therefore, some loss of fine detail is experienced (3). A Kodachrome slide, for example, can show a particular image in great detail, but because videotape involves motion, the detail obtained is not as great.

While videotape can be misused as a teaching-learning resource, it can also be a very effective medium for teachers and students. With it, a particular program can be distributed electronically from one station to another, providing instant, simultaneous viewing for more than one group of students. A well-prepared teacher can thus reach more students than could normally be accommodated in an ordinary classroom.

Videotape is one means by which the quality of instruction can be maintained, or even improved, when teachers are faced with increased enrollments but no increase in faculty and staff. Many types of subject content or procedures can be taught as effectively through use of videotape as through conventional (face-to-face) demonstrations (17). Specific laboratory or clinical procedures can be prerecorded on videotape, for example, and played back during class with the teacher narrating particular aspects. In this instance a class session that formerly had to be spent with many small groups, because close, at-hand student observation was required, can now be conducted with a large

---

*From J. W. Brown et al., *AV Instruction: Technology, Media, and Methods,* 5th ed. (New York: McGraw-Hill, © 1977), p. 75. Used with permission of McGraw-Hill Book Company.

group of students. Although extra effort is initially required of the teacher to produce the recordings, a considerable net savings of time and energy is possible, since the videotape can be reused until the procedures are revised.

Three general *purposes* can be served through use of videotape: to demonstrate procedures, depict situations, or present patients.

Procedures can be demonstrated in several ways with videotape. A commercial or locally produced tape can demonstrate an entire procedure, with a voice-over explaining in detail what is occurring. This type of tape could be used in class or put on reserve in a library or resource center for individual student use. Another tape may include the demonstration only, without narration; the teacher could use this as an in-class resource much like a chalkboard or slide projector, supplying personal commentary and stopping and restarting the tape when necessary. In either instance, students would subsequently be given the opportunity to practice the procedure in a laboratory setting until they can successfully perform it themselves.

Students can easily learn to operate videotape equipment, particularly the portable models, and they can take turns taping each other performing procedures in front of the camera. Here the videotape would be used for demonstrating a procedure; it would also provide students the opportunity for self-evaluation, as well as for peer teaching, if they meet in small groups to critique each other's tapes.

Videotapes can be used to present vignettes of real or simulated behaviors, events, or patient-care situations. Vignettes can be used in class to stimulate discussions, to demonstrate effective or ineffective ways of dealing with particular situations, or to illustrate the consequences of a health-care professional's behavior. In these instances they can be very effective in contributing to the achievement of learning objectives that involve verbal and nonverbal communication, interpersonal interaction, or attitude formation (14).

Sometimes one vignette can be used by several departments or courses as a resource associated with a variety of objectives. For example, a vignette could depict a closed psychiatric unit of 25 patients, some of them acutely disturbed, in which a resident, a nurse, and two aides are on duty one evening. Role playing by performers would be involved here, so the vignette needs to be larger than life in order to be as provocative and attention-getting as possible. The person playing the lead role, a disturbed patient, first encourages another patient to eat one of the plastic ornaments off the Christmas tree, and then sneaks off to use the telephone (inadvertently left on) to order twelve dozen pairs of nylons for his wife. As the nurse begins to deal with this situation, a call comes from the lobby: 15 pizzas have arrived for the patient and the pizza man wants his money.

This vignette could be used with student nurses to analyze the behavior patterns of a manic depressive patient. Or, it could be used to help aides anticipate the kinds of ward behaviors they may be asked to respond to in actual settings. It could also be used to help medical students beginning a rotation to anticipate ward management problems and to become familiar with potential interpersonal and interprofessional dynamics of a ward.

Another form of vignette can be used to present patients to students at the most appropriate or convenient time. It often happens that a patient with a certain disorder is in a clinic or hospital at a time when no students are scheduled to study the disorder. In most cases the teacher must then decide whether to change the teaching plan or simply refer back to this particular patient sometime later in the course or unit. Neither of these options has yet provided very satisfactory results. By videotaping the examination, diagnosis, or procedures called for, however, the teacher can have the patient available whenever necessary.

This kind of vignette can also be effective in helping students develop their communication skills. Actual professional-patient interactions can be shown outside the clinical setting, so that students can observe and begin developing a repertoire of behaviors for later use. With the aid of videotape, students can experiment with priority making, decision making, and assessment skills before they actually work in clinical settings.

Because of the availability of videotapes on a wide range of subjects, teachers are often able to purchase a tape for use in their courses. As many videotapes as possible should be previewed to determine their suitability to specific learning objectives. Many times an externally produced tape will be appropriate to objectives and subject content; in these instances, the tape should be purchased to avoid later internal production of essentially the same material. Sometimes, however, none of the videotapes previewed is suitable, particularly when the purpose for using a tape is extremely specific. In these instances, one has to be produced. The good and bad points noted of the previewed tapes then serve to guide the teacher's own production. The teacher must consider all possible production costs and then develop a reasonable *production budget*.

There are very few satisfactory general formulas for establishing a production budget. Budgets will vary significantly, depending on the sophistication of the intended tape and on whether its purpose is to demonstrate a procedure, depict situations, or present patients. They will also vary according to the resources that are available for use. Some institutions have media staff and specialists in various phases of production who usually become involved from the very beginning in the production of instructional media and follow a project through to its completion. Other schools have available for assistance to teachers the use of studios and production facilities, as well as technician time. Still others have very few of these resources, so that interested teachers have to do everything for themselves, including writing the script, running the camera, and editing for a final copy. The purpose to be fulfilled by a teacher-produced videotape, its level of sophistication, and its budget requirements will therefore be dictated in part by the nature of available production facilities and equipment.

Many schools have elaborate libraries or learning resource centers with video and audio equipment, while others may need to purchase equipment. If the teacher becomes involved in purchasing videotape equipment, some caution is necessary. Currently, standardization of videotapes is still something of a problem, as there are formats for 1-inch, 2-inch, 3½-inch, and disk videotapes. Any selection of a tape format should be made in light of other formats currently in use or projected for use by other departments or units of the institution.

At a basic level, equipment purchased should be simple to operate and yet able to meet existing and potential needs. If it is intended primarily for student use in a laboratory, for example, a portable camera-recording unit would be sufficient. If the teacher wants sophisticated productions, studio equipment and expert consultation are needed. Both teachers and schools should not invest large sums of money in purchasing expensive equipment, however, and then be obligated to artificially stimulate faculty interest to justify the expense. It is ultimately a sounder policy to produce simple videotapes and use the money saved to provide faculty release time for additional special educational projects or course development.

Approaches to *producing* a videotape can vary as much as production budgets, and for the same reasons. Teachers whose schools or departments have access to production facilities will already have one or more approaches to choose from. Teachers with no such facilities immediately available should consult as many resource persons and materials as possible when considering production possibilities (see the Unit 2 bibliography).

The basic approach to producing a videotape entails first outlining the content to be presented, so that an overview of its parts is developed. This overview highlights the main content elements of the intended presentation and suggests the ordering of information within each element. The main content elements initially suggest the structure, flow, and pace of the production; they later become production segments that are taped and combined to form a finished videotape.

A storyboard of the production follows, along with the development of a script that details the content presentation to be made. A storyboard is developed by writing production notes on separate index cards; these indicate what the audience should be hearing and observing for each main content element (e.g., "close-up of schizophrenic patient, voiceover of resident psychiatrist"). A rough draft, and later a refined version of the script, indicate what the audience will be hearing; sketches or rough stick-figure drawings, accompanied by appropriate camera directions, indicate what they will be seeing. After revision and refinement, the storyboard is made into a shooting script, used to direct the actual taping. Because one advantage of videotape is its erasable quality, the actual taping of each production segment can be done at least twice, with critiques after each taping, so that the final product is satisfactory to the teacher and effective for the student.

Slide-tapes

A slide-tape presentation is a motionless multimedia form consisting of simultaneous verbal and visual messages. It allows students to listen to a presentation while watching slides that illustrate its major points. When well-planned and executed, the verbal and visual messages of a slide-tape complement each other to create a stronger impact than either alone (11).

Slide-tape presentations can be very elaborate, involving material and devices that periodically ask the student a question, and then, according to the response, go forward or return to an appropriate point and rerun the program. They can also be very simple and straightforward, presenting graphs, charts, drawings, or photographs to illustrate subject content.

Teachers interested in including a slide-tape in a course, after first determining that it would be an appropriate media form for specific learning objectives and deciding how it might best be used, should first find out what is available for purchase by consulting the sources previously discussed.

If nothing appropriate or acceptable is found, the prospects of producing a slide-tape can be considered. Unlike a videotape, whose quality increases in proportion to the amount of money, technical assistance, and production facilities available, a good slide-tape can be produced by teachers themselves, with varying degrees of assistance. Like a videotape, production of a slide-tape begins with the formulation of a *budget*. The budget should estimate not only the expenditure of financial resources, but also the expenditure of the teacher's time.

Until teachers prepare a script and know what kind of visuals, graphics, artwork, and line photography shots will be needed, costs will be difficult to estimate. If any kind of future distribution is being considered, original visuals are usually suggested. Thus, an artist may be needed to prepare some of the materials, while teachers may be able to do some artwork themselves. A photographer may also be a necessity, although teachers should not be afraid to take their own pictures. Some fine slides have been made with inexpensive, easy-to-operate cameras, especially those equipped with tripods or stands that hold the camera still.

The financial costs involved in producing a slide-tape can include the time of a professional photographer or artist, the cost of film and audiotape, and the cost of graphic materials. They can also include the allocation of equipment needed to use the slide-tape in a course. Study carrels in an instructional-materials center or library provide for optimum student use of slide-tapes. If these facilities are unavailable, an improvised carrel in a quiet room can be constructed using a wall as the screen and a table holding the slide projector, earphones, and a small tape recorder.

Estimating equipment costs is difficult; a reasonable figure often depends on availability. How much is needed for ten, thirty, or sixty students can be calculated only when it is known if the equipment to be used will be available for, say, three hours a day twice a week, or ten hours a day seven days a week. Media resources and appropriate equipment are usually kept in a library or resource center, but some schools find it helpful to keep copies and a study carrel in laboratories or hospital units, so that students who like to study late at night or at unusual times may do so. In planning to use slide-tapes, then, the teacher needs to estimate equipment costs not only on the basis of the number of students who will use the resource but also on the basis of the times the resource will be available to them.

The expenditure of a teacher's time will depend on how comfortable the teacher feels with the content material to be presented by the slide-tape. For example, a teacher may consider using a slide-tape for a difficult lecture, one for which problems have already been identified. In this case, time will be spent reviewing and revising the content and organization of the original presentation. On the other hand, a teacher planning to produce a slide-tape on material that is already well defined, perhaps through current lecture notes, will have half the preparatory work already done.

In either case, the first slide-tape script a teacher attempts will take longer to develop and write than later ones. It may take a month to write the script, for example, and another month or longer to produce the program; teachers need to allow for this. While it may seem hard to fit the first slide-tape script into a busy teaching schedule, time and experience will show that it can take less time to prepare a script than a lecture.

The teacher begins *production* of a slide-tape much as if preparing for a lecture. By going to the library and reading what ordinarily would constitute the parts of a student assignment, the teacher seeks out several sources and selects appropriate information from each. Material is therefore brought together from a variety of sources and edited to fit the conceptual framework and time limitations of the intended slide-tape presentation. By using the finished slide-tape, students will not have to search for and read several reference sources to get the one or two paragraphs the teacher thinks are most important.

After gathering the material, the teacher begins to write the script using a form similar to that shown in Fig. 5.1. Major points to be made in the slide-tape are first identified, then written down in narrative form. Each point or idea should be limited to a maximum of about three sentences; one idea follows another in sequence down the left-hand side of the page. When this writing process is completed, the entire draft is read through to make sure it contains exactly what is intended. Because the script will eventually be heard and not read, it is very helpful to tape-record a reading of the script and then listen to it. Since paragraphs, italics, and similar written conventions have no

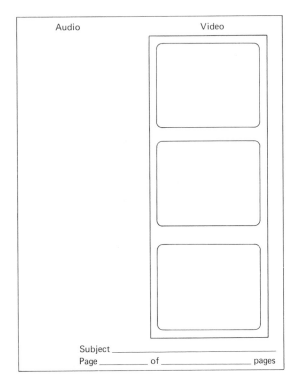

Fig. 5.1
Script flowchart for slide-tape production.

meaning in an audio production, it is important that the script sound clear to the listener.

With a draft of the script on the left side of the form, the teacher can begin to add corresponding visuals on the right side. At this stage, a sketch is sufficient, using stick figures or drawings.

There are several types of visuals. Photographs or artists' drawings are used to illustrate the general concepts covered in the narration and usually comprise the basic visual material of the whole presentation. Graphs and diagrams can make statistics and technical information much clearer and easier to understand. The diagram or graph should be simple, however, avoiding small detail when possible. If detail is important, that information can be provided by a sequence of slides showing progressively more detail. Word visuals, used by themselves or superimposed on photographs or drawings, focus attention on central ideas and help to establish relationships. Only key words or central ideas or relationships should be used, however, to avoid later problems of readability (4).

Pacing in a slide-tape presentation is crucial and is established initially when visuals are matched with segments of the script. Pacing, a quality specific to each slide-tape, depends on the nature of the content, visuals, and narration selected. Proper pacing is achieved when the coordinated verbal and visual messages proceed in a fashion that allows both the general and specific ideas of the slide-tape to be received and understood. Although a highly individualistic characteristic, its success can be ensured in part by mixing art with photography, varying the time each visual frame is on the screen, and using sequence shots or close-ups to accompany long narrative segments.

Once production of the unit begins, the sketched-out artwork and photography need to be completed. Several photos should be shot of everything; film is inexpensive compared to the time and material resources the teacher has invested up to this point. Though the audiotape is often recorded in a sound studio, a quiet room and inexpensive tape-recorder may be quite adequate. Male voices usually project better than female voices if inexpensive equipment must be used.

After the unit has been prepared, a content expert should review the script for inaccuracies. Mistakes can be made when the teacher is attempting to present content in a condensed form, for it is easier to present total content in minute detail than it is to select essentials and present them consistently. The ability to distinguish the essential from the supplementary, and to present it effectively, is the test of any teacher.

If the slide-tape program is for the beginning student, a lay person or colleague not familiar with the content should take a pretest, view the slide-tape, and then take a posttest. If the program is for advanced students, someone with the same background and degree of knowledge ultimately expected of the students viewing the program should do the same thing. From this testing, the teacher will be able to determine if any prerequisites for the unit are needed. Some teachers build lectures on knowledge they assume their students already possess, only to find the students do not have it. This assumption can be carried over to the development of slide-tape programs. If some prerequisites are needed, it is wise to include them with the written materials prepared to accompany the slide-tape.

Audiotapes

Audiotapes are verbal media, generally used as alternatives to the printed text. They can be effective additions to a teacher's fund of media resources, particularly for use with students who have some reading difficulty (16), for they communicate more vividly and with greater feeling than can a text.

The major *purpose* of audiotapes is documentary in nature—preserving conversations, discussions, or other verbal activities for use as teaching tools. To this end, audiotapes can be used at the bedside of patients to help students develop their communication skills. A recording of a student's verbal interaction with a patient, for example, can form the basis for the student's self-critique of the conversation and the communication principles involved. The teacher can evaluate the student's progress in the area by first listening to the tape, then reading the self-critique, and finally discussing the process and its results with the student.

Audiotaped vignettes can be used in much the same way as videotapes to stimulate group discussion. If the topic is drug abuse, for example, and students have already done enough preparatory work to be able to discuss incidents, symptoms, and treatment, an audiotape vignette of a nurse-addict can be an effective teaching-learning device. The vignette, which should include two or more speakers to add variety and allow flexibility in the presentation, might consist of a "head nurse" confronting a "nurse-addict" to illustrate the difficulty of dealing with a professional suspected of drug abuse. Like the videotape, the audiotape can be stopped at various points to raise or clarify issues or to call for the application of previously learned content.

Audiotapes have frequently been used to tape-record lectures, either for absent students or for a permanent record of the lecture for future use. While it is sometimes necessary to record a lecture for students, the proper use of audiotapes does not include the routine taping of lectures, for it diminishes any incentive to change the lecture for subsequent presentations. Further, a tape-recorded lecture tends to be boring, even confusing, if the lecturer has made use of the chalkboard or other visuals. Thus, if for some reason a lecture must be recorded, it should be edited to omit these and similar occurrences and to ensure that only the speaker's main points are included.

Audiotapes are easy to produce and are considerably less expensive than videotapes. Major *budget* considerations focus on the type of format used in the institution, i.e., reel-to-reel, cassette, or cartridge, so that standardization is maintained when tapes are purchased. The number of tapes to be reproduced and the manner in which they are duplicated also must be considered in developing a budget. Equipment for playing audiotapes can be very inexpensive. If a tape-recorder is to be used also with slide-tape programs, it will receive more wear and therefore should be heavier and of better quality than the typical portable models.

Plans for *production* of this media form begin with an assessment of the material the audiotape is intended to accompany—i.e., what type and level of learning objectives are involved? If the objectives involve interaction and deal with cognitive or affective content, an audiotape can be an appropriate medium to use in conjunction with them (6). The basic production process followed is then similar to that of a videotape. The teacher begins by developing a storyboard and a script detailing the content presentation, but omits the graphics. Actual production is much simpler than that of a videotape; the main concern is to procure a quiet room or area for recording, so that extraneous noise is deleted or at least minimized.

Transparencies for Overhead Projection

Transparencies for overhead projection represent a versatile alternative to the chalkboard. They provide the means for presenting a variety of types of images in a range of sizes, colors, and special effects. While the chalkboard limits the scope and design of a teacher's visual presentation (one that accompanies a lecture, for example), overhead transparencies are limited only by a teacher's creativity and time commitment and by the resources available for purchasing or producing them.

Overhead projection of transparencies differs from previously discussed media forms in that its use is usually confined to the classroom and requires the presence of a teacher. Unlike some visual media, such as slides or film, transparencies for overhead projection can be used in a lighted room, thus facilitating student note taking or reference to other materials. They can also be modified extemporaneously or saved for reuse at a later time.

The major *purpose* of overhead transparencies is to provide a source of content or to support or illustrate the content of a teacher's lecture presentation while allowing the teacher to maintain face-to-face contact with the class of students. A teacher can use transparencies to present a complete outline at the outset of a lecture, for example, to provide an overview of what is to come, or to fill in an incomplete outline as the lecture presentation progresses. Actual objects such as syringe needles, catheter tubes, or asepto syringes may be placed on the overhead projector and then be discussed or demonstrated with the benefit of magnification. Transparencies can also be developed to present pictures, diagrams, graphs, charts, or other illustrative material singly or in sequence using overlays. In addition, by attaching plastic, light-polarizing materials to the surface of a transparency, a teacher can produce motion effects to illustrate such factors as circulation, respiration, or fluid movements.

Budget considerations associated with overhead transparencies depend on whether the transparencies are purchased or produced. The costs of commercially prepared transparencies may vary somewhat from company to company, but generally are proportionate to the amount of technical sophistication, complexity, or special effects afforded a particular transparency. Because a considerable array of these materials is available for purchase, the teacher should first consult media catalogues to compare content, display techniques, and costs.

The costs of teacher-made transparencies are largely determined by the type of production method chosen. Basically, there are three ways teachers can easily *produce* a transparency. The most common, and the least expensive, is the direct process method in which a colored felt pen, wax pencil, or typewriter is used to imprint an image on a piece of clear acetate material. This method most closely approximates writing on a chalkboard and is appropriate when single-dimension visuals are needed, e.g., verbal information, tables, graphs. Costs here involve only acetate material and writing instruments.

Two other common production methods, both of which allow for the development of elaborate transparencies, are the heat-transfer and the diazo processes. The heat-transfer process is the simpler and involves transferring original materials to transparency form through use of a thermographic machine, such as a Thermo-Fax copy machine. The diazo process, used to develop permanent color transparencies, entails processing exposed diazo film in ammonia vapor. Neither method requires extensive technical preparation by teachers; those interested in producing their own transparencies need only the proper equipment, supplies, and patience. Costs depend on the degree of complexity or sophistication of the planned transparencies, the materials to be used, and the type of equipment available. Both methods are also commonly used by technical staffs associated with media resource centers or illustration-photography departments. The costs of either will thus be established by the production unit whose services are available to the teacher.

Programmed Instruction

Programmed instruction is a general approach to developing materials students can use to achieve specific minimal competence objectives. The teacher's *purpose* in programming materials is to divide subject content into a series of small, discrete parts. These parts are presented in such a way as to require an active response from students; any response is followed by some form of feedback, which contributes to the way subsequent responses are given (7).

The product of the programming process may be presented through any one of several media forms, e.g., workbooks, teaching machines, computers, or slide-tapes, which in turn may or may not utilize a variety of supportive materials, such as physical models, films, or videotapes. The medium chosen will be an active carrier of learning conditions, for it will provide opportunities for students to practice specific behaviors and receive continuous feedback and reinforcement on their progress. These generalized conditions can follow either a linear pattern, in which subject content is arranged in a series of steps progressing in a single direction, or a branching pattern, in which each step encountered presents several alternatives, so that a variety of directions through the subject content is possible.

The development of even the simplest linear program can be time consuming; more elaborate, branching programs require patience, experience, and, in most cases, technical assistance. Teachers interested in the teaching-learning applications of programmed instruction might best be advised to acquire commercial or externally produced materials when beginning their investigations in this area. The examination, selection, and use of published materials not only helps teachers become familiar with the concept and function of programmed instruction, it can also provide the foundation teachers need to produce their own programs.

As with any other media resource, *budget* considerations frequently play a part in the selection and use of programmed-instruction materials. The costs associated with published materials vary according to the sophistication of the program and the medium used to present it. A linear program dealing with basic statistical concepts and presented in workbook form can be available at typical paperback-book prices. A computerized branching program dealing with clinical problem solving may cost several thousand dollars to acquire and make ready for student use. Costs can also vary among publishers; materials produced by another school are likely to be less expensive than those produced by a commercial publishing house.

Aside from considerations of cost, several other criteria should be used in evaluating programmed instructional materials (1). These criteria can be stated as questions the teacher should answer while examining specific programs:

1. Have the *objectives* for the program been established on the basis of an adequate task analysis? Must the student demonstrate specific behaviors or skills directly relevant to some real-world task that must eventually be performed?

2. What is the *nature of the responses called for*? Do the responses require active thought, or merely the copying of words or phrases previously provided? Do they assist or interfere with the student's focus of attention? Are the responses immediately related to the critical structure of the subject, or to small, irrelevant bits of the overall structure?

3. Does the *organization and sequencing* used in the program reflect an adequate behavior analysis? Is information presented so as to build appropriate thought patterns? Are categories and pieces of information presented to the student at the time in the program when they are truly needed? Are they presented in a manner that allows students to apply the information to the performance of required tasks?

Answers to these questions necessitate a knowledge of the structure of the subject content being programmed. They also require a familiarity with the associationist learning principles underlying programmed instruction.

Teachers interested in the *production* of their own programmed materials, yet who feel they lack the time or expertise needed for traditional linear or branching programs, should consider the development of adjunct programs. An adjunct program utilizes preexisting materials, such as texts, journal articles, media resources, X-rays, or physical models, to provide subject content. It also includes teacher-made instructions, practice exercises, and question-and-answer sequences that provide direction for student progress through the program. The teacher's contribution thus represents an addition to traditional materials that unifies and focuses them for students' independent study toward specific objectives.

The development of an adjunct program begins with identification of the objectives students are to achieve on their own when provided with appropriate materials. As the program will provide an alternative to a lecture or discussion session, the teacher's primary development task is to create a set of instructions and question-and-answer sequences that will direct students through the materials to the objectives. The teacher first determines which sections of texts, journal articles, or other resources will be essential for students' attainment of objectives. The resources are then arranged in a logical sequence that forms the beginning, middle, and end of the students' confrontation with content related to the objectives. With this sequence arranged, the teacher engages in mental dialogues with advanced, average, and slow students, taking each type through the content with a question-and-answer approach. These "dialogues" will be based on prior experiences with students of each type and will help the teacher formulate both the actual questions and the different feedback responses that will later guide students through the materials.

When a set of instructions and question-and-answer sequences have been written, the adjunct program is ready to be pilot-tested. To ensure that the teacher has accurately anticipated the reactions of students of different abilities, the pilot test is conducted with students whose backgrounds and educational levels are similar to those of the students who will eventually use the program. The pilot students should be asked to work through the program to its conclusion, respond to a posttest referenced to the program's objectives, and evaluate the program in terms of such factors as the amount of time required, the clarity of the instructions, and the appropriateness of the amount of material contained in the program.

REFERENCES

1. ADLER, JACK H. "Intrinsic Criteria for the Evaluation of a Medical Program." In Jerome P. Lysaught, ed., *Instructional Systems in Medical Education*. New York: The Rochester Clearinghouse, University of Rochester, 1970, pp. 137–145.

2. ALLEN, WILLIAM H. "Intellectual Abilities and Instructional Media Design." *AV Communication Review* 23 (Summer 1975): 139–170.

3. ALLEN, WILLIAM J. "Media Stimulus and Types of Learning." In *Selecting Media for Learning*. Washington, D.C.: Association for Educational Communications and Technology, 1974, pp. 8–12.

4. BROWN, JAMES W., RICHARD B. LEWIS, AND FRED F. HARCLEROAD. *AV Instruction: Technology, Media, and Methods*. 5th ed. New York: McGraw-Hill, 1977.

5. CAMPEAU, PEGGIE L. "Selective Review of the Results of Research on the Use of Audiovisual Media to Teach Adults." *AV Communication Review* 16 (Spring 1974): 5–40.

6. EDLING, JACK V. "Educational Objectives and Educational Media." *Review of Educational Research* 38 (April 1968): 177–194.

7. GREEN, EDWARD J. *The Learning Process and Programmed Instruction.* New York: Holt, Rinehart, and Winston, 1962.

8. GROPPER, GEORGE L. "A Behavioral Perspective on Media Selection." *AV Communication Review* 24 (Summer 1976): 157–186.

9. McCONNELL, JOHN TERENCE. "If the Medium Fits, Use It!" In *Selecting Media for Learning.* Washington, D.C.: Association for Educational Communications and Technology, 1974, pp. 22–26.

10. MINOR, ED, AND HARVEY R. FRYE. *Techniques for Producing Visual Instructional Material.* 2d ed. New York: McGraw-Hill, 1977.

11. NASSER, DAVID L., AND WILLIAM J. McEWEN. "The Impact of Alternative Media Channels: Recall and Involvement with Messages." *AV Communication Review* 24 (Fall 1976): 263–272.

12. NATIONAL INFORMATION CENTER FOR EDUCATIONAL MEDIA. *Index to Health and Safety Education (Multimedia).* Los Angeles: University of Southern California.

13. NATIONAL MEDICAL AUDIOVISUAL CENTER. *Catalogue of Audiovisuals for the Health Scientist.* U.S. Department of Health, Education, and Welfare, Public Health Service, National Institutes of Health, National Library of Medicine, National Medical Audiovisual Center, Atlanta, Georgia, 1974, with supplementary listings.

14. RAMEY, JAMES W. "Self-Instructional Uses of Television in Health Science Education." In Jerome P. Lysaught, ed. *Instructional Systems in Medical Education*, New York: The Rochester Clearinghouse, University of Rochester, 1970, pp. 93–100.

15. ROGERS, CARL R. *Freedom to Learn.* Columbus, Ohio: Merrill, 1969.

16. SNOW, R. E., AND G. SALOMON. "Aptitudes and Instructional Media." *AV Communication Review* 16 (1968): 341–357.

17. TOMETSKO, ANDREW M. "Curriculum Flexibility and Independent Study in Medical Education." In Jerome P. Lysaught, ed., *Instructional Technology in Medical Education.* New York: The Rochester Clearinghouse, University of Rochester, 1973, pp. 141–150.

6
SIMULATION GAMES

Simulations are simplified reality: they represent the essence of physical or social systems of interaction. Simulations attempt to replicate essential aspects of reality, so that reality may be better understood and/or controlled. Hence, something *out there* is to be modeled *here* (15).

Physical simulations are based on a model of some object, e.g., a model of the cardiovascular system demonstrating blood flow under different conditions. Social simulations deal with people and, therefore, are based on a model of some facet of a social system or institution, e.g., the professional and patient community of a family practice clinic. Social simulations used for educational purposes entail individuals or groups of individuals assuming and acting out specific roles representing those of the real world. These simulations are usually presented in the format of a game (12).

A game is an activity undertaken by players whose actions are limited to a set of explicit rules particular to that activity and by a predetermined, artificial stopping point. A game provides competitive interaction among participants to achieve prespecified goals. This interaction may feature cooperation within groups, but competition either among individuals or groups distinguishes gaming from other exercises (15). A game is usually played for entertainment and is intended to have clearly identified winners and losers; participant success is dependent on skill or chance or some combination of the two. A game makes no attempt to replicate real-world behavior—rules of behavior for the game need apply to the game only.

From these two ideas—simulation to represent elements of reality and gaming to encourage interaction—a variety of powerful learning activities commonly known as educational simulation games have been developed.

Participants in a simulation game interact within an artificially produced environment designed to represent some aspect of an actual social system. They assume roles and the particular goals of the individuals or groups being simulated and conduct themselves in the context of specific rules. Participants experience success or failure in a manner similar to their real-world counterparts, depending on how strategies are planned and available resources used (12).

Simulation games differ from the simulation exercises developed to assess students' problem-solving abilities (see Chapter 13). The latter type of simulation is precisely programmed according to the history and personality of the patient simulated, so that nothing is left to chance (11). Student response alternatives are highly structured, so that, for example, response F will automatically be followed by alternative G. Such inflexible structure is not characteristic of social simulation games.

FUNCTIONS OF SIMULATION GAMES

Simulation games can be used in many ways to facilitate the achievement of different types of learning objectives. They can be used to motivate students, since they involve active participation by the student in what can be an enjoyable experience. They can aid in the acquisition and retention of factual knowledge, help to form or change attitudes (9), provide an opportunity for students to acquire and practice social skills, and be used to evaluate student performance (15).

There are several advantages to including simulation games in the teaching-learning process. Simulations provide a relatively safe but standardized learning environment. Students can be less concerned about harming a patient and pleasing the teacher and can concentrate on learning. Since the simulated environment is standardized, teachers' attempts at evaluating student performance can be more consistent. In addition, the fact that learning and assessment tasks are preselected means that they can be carefully increased in difficulty as students progress through an educational program. In effect, by developing standard, parallel simulations, it is possible to confront students over and over again with interesting variations in what is essentially the same task until they have mastered it. Simulation games also enable the teacher to standardize the task for all students, and, in the case of such things as medical examinations, to do so without subjecting one or a few patients to repeated bombardment by a large number of students.

One of the most important advantages of simulation games over reality is the fact that all students can be allowed full responsibility for their own behavior without risk to anyone. This is important, particularly for the type of self-directed professional education advocated in this book. For example, a student can be allowed to continue along an ill-considered or incorrect course and receive realistic feedback without harm to anyone. A simulated patient can become progressively sicker, die, commit suicide, or leave the clinic, and yet be repeatedly "revived" to confront the same or other students.

Simulation games are not only interesting in themselves, they serve to provoke further student interest in subject matter, particularly for underachieving students or those with inadequately developed verbal skills (1). Consequently, because of their motivation value, some teachers schedule games at the start of a unit in order to arouse class interest.

Simulation games can be used to accommodate a variety of learning styles. Students who respond poorly to traditional methods of teaching may respond quite well to simulation learning experiences. Because there is no relationship between the standard academic achievement of the student and the student's game performance (14), a student who does poorly in a typical classroom situation in which verbal and conceptual skills are required may do exceptionally well in a simulation game, even when reading and writing skills are essential. It is not clear why this occurs. Since games use interactive skills, however, they may not be as threatening to the poorer student (5) or may appeal to some students who prefer to learn through interactive experiences. Whatever the reason, games provide an opportunity for enactive learning—the kind of learning that takes place when someone performs a task correctly and knows it is correct, even if unable to say why. Students who are still struggling to achieve competence with verbal skills learn, on an enactive level, if given the opportunity (2).

Simulation games also provide an opportunity for experiential learning—the kind of learning in which students experience some of the doubts, difficulties, and anxieties they would experience in the actual clinical interchange. This type of learning seems to stay with the student longer than does information processing (16). In the latter, the student receives information via lecture or book, arrives at an understanding of the general and then particular application, and then acts. In experiential learning, such as simulation gaming, the student acts first, then begins to understand how to apply principles and concepts, and later has a chance to act again in a different (sometimes real-life) situation (4). Since experiential learning can stay with the student longer, and because simulation gaming can teach factual information as well as other methods of instruction (13), health science teachers need to evaluate the balance between information processing and experiential learning that exists in some courses.

Finally, many students prefer simulation games to other types of classroom activities. This, of course, has implications for teaching students with low levels of motivation. Teachers with such students need to consider these activities as possible alternate learning experiences.

Simulation games also have several disadvantages. In some professions, for example, there are very few simulation games on the market; the many good simulation games developed by schools or departments are frequently not widely known or readily obtained. Many of the commercially prepared materials available are not well designed. As a result, students do not learn apropriate behaviors or experience desired changes in attitudes. Finally, the development and use of simulation games is time consuming. A teacher needs only several minutes to tell students what kind of emotional reactions to expect from a dying patient, while to develop and use a simulation game that allows students to experience at least some aspect of working with a dying patient takes much longer. Some teachers may not think the trade-off in time is worthwhile.

Many teachers may feel uncomfortable with the simulation game format of teaching-learning, since it is unfamiliar to them. While simulation games encourage academic achievement as effectively as more traditional controlled teaching strategies, such as lectures (7), teachers sometimes intuitively feel that students cannot be learning properly if they seem to be having fun. A teacher who is unwilling to devote sufficient time to the selection and preparation of simulation games, or who feels more comfortable and secure in the standard lecture format, will find the use of simulation games difficult and frustrating. Furthermore, in some instances, a lecture on a topic may be more pointed and more beneficial to students than a simulation game concerning the same topic.

A final word of caution: Simulation games "imitate," they do not "duplicate" real life. Clearly, some things cannot be simulated. To predict how a student will behave in actual situations is not possible; it is only possible to predict how a student is "capable" of behaving.

TYPES OF SIMULATION GAMES

A teacher considering the possible use of simulation gaming activities should reexamine the minimal and the developmental competence objectives that have already been established. Both levels of objectives, whether cognitive or attitudinal, can be approached by students engaged in simulation games.

There are four broad categories of simulation games: nonsimulation games, planning exercises, interpersonal simulation games, and large-system simulation games (15).

The first category, *nonsimulation games*, is composed of competitive learning situations in which participant success is determined by the degree of subject matter comprehension—of information, concepts, generalizations, and/or theories—that is demonstrated during game play.

- *Example:* A card game called "guts" is developed to teach the physiology of digestion (10). The game is based on rummy and can be used for practice and reinforcement as well as some initial learning. Points are allocated in this game and the highest score at the end of the time is the winner.

Planning exercises focus on process rather than content by engaging the participant in the examination of selected social problems requiring solution. Committees cooperate in discussion and each proposes a solution, which is judged by the entire group after evaluation criteria have been established and applied.

- *Example:*   A teacher wishes to help students plan total patient care, recognize priorities of care, and gain insight into ward management. A board game is devised so that the patient's progress from the "start" (admission) through to the "finish" (discharge), is controlled by the throw of die and selection of instruction cards. It enables a group of learners to see how both careful and haphazard planning affects patient care and length of stay in the hospital.

Interpersonal simulation games provide learning situations in which participants respond as if they were in the actual system of interaction being modeled. Rules and physical circumstances structure the interactions, producing interactions ranging from the highly restricted participant behavior of a computer-simulated game through the less inhibited behavior associated with a "board game" to the flexible, open-ended behavior of role-playing simulation games. The latter most closely approximates the actual system of interaction being simulated.

Interpersonal simulation games combine the aspects of gaming with the reality replication of simulation to allow the participant a personal glimpse of how it "feels" to be involved in interpersonal interactions. This category can also include use of media-based training exercises, communication-skills exercises, and the wide range of exercises and activities developed for human-relations training.

- *Example:*   "A Day in Ward 10" is a simulation for groups of nurses who take on the roles of nurses, patients, relatives, and other hospital personnel (10). Crises are introduced on a programmed basis, requiring each group to make decisions simultaneously within a stated time. The decision of each group is discussed and rated according to various criteria, such as communication skills and sensitivity.

Large-system simulation games are learning situations that enable the examination of the dynamics of complex systems of interaction. Participants engage in all aspects of the simulated system—in planning, decision making, and observing—in order to better understand some of the variables affecting human behavior within the context of the actual complex system being simulated.

- *Example:*   "Synoptics" is a game designed to help health professionals view the delivery of health care from various perspectives (5). The game creates a milieu favorable to the discussion of how health-care issues can be seen from a variety of perspectives. The game is structured by assigning roles to twelve players and dividing them into three groups. The three groups are presented with a problem situation and are asked to respond to it. Each of the groups is a "patient-care committee" of City Hospital. Other players are asked to be members of a jury. They are told to deliberate and then vote to determine which of the three groups generated the best response to the problem. After this group has been identified, all of the participants engage in a debriefing or follow-up discussion session.

The effectiveness ratings of the four general categories of simulation games, given in Table 6.1 in terms of specific characteristics, can be used as one approach to the selection of a simulation gaming activity that would be most appropriate for specific learning objectives.

Table 6.1.
A Comparison of Simulation/Gaming Applications[7]

Scale: 1 = Low in characteristic
        5 = High in characteristic

Characteristic	Nonsimulation Game	Planning Exercise	Interpersonal Simulation Game	Large-System Simulation Game
1. Dependability of learning outcomes	3	2	2	4
2. Ease of adaption	5	4	3	1
3. Degree of teacher centeredness	1	3	3	3
4. Degree of complexity and exposure	1	2	2–3	5
5. Peer interaction	4	4	5	1–3
6. Focus on interpersonal and social processes	2	2	5	3
7. Accommodate heterogeneous groups	5	4	4	3
8. Peer feedback/ evaluation	5	4	4	2–4
9. Ease of accommodation of various size groups	4	5	3	4
10. Ease of insertion into curriculum	5	5	4	3
11. Cognitive learning outcomes				
A. Facts	5	4	3	5
B. Concepts	5	4	3	4
C. Generalizations	5	4	3	4

Table 6.1 (cont'd)

Characteristic	Nonsimulation Game	Planning Exercise	Interpersonal Simulation Game	Large-System Simulation Game
D. Principles	5	3	3	5
E. Drawing analogies	1	3	4	5
F. Identifying strategies	1	3–4	4	5
G. Extrapolating from data	1	4	3	5
H. Interpretation	1	4	4	5
I. Application	1	5	4	4
J. Analysis	1	4	4	5
K. Synthesis	1	4	4	5
L. Evaluation	1	4	4	5
12. Affective learning outcomes				
A. Involvement	5	5	5	5
B. Emotion exhibited	5	3	5	3
C. Perception of others	2	3	5	2
D. Perception of self	3	3	5	3
E. Sense of control	3	3	5	3
F. Attitude toward				
1. Subject	5	5	5	5
2. Instructor	5	5	5	5
3. Peers (playing)	5	4	5	4
G. Motivation to participate	5	4	5	4
H. Level of inter-actions among participants	5	5	5	5

On a general level, the activities included in each of these categories can be used successfully with a variety of students who have a variety of backgrounds and interests. On a specific level, it has been suggested that students who derive maximum benefit from simulation gaming activities are likely to be those who (a) gather a great deal of information from listening to others; (b) derive meaning from sounds other than words or numbers; (c) empathize; (d) prefer peer-group interaction; (e) can, but do not prefer to, operate in independent-study settings; and (f) reason to some degree through the application of rules and/or definitions

(6). Thus, when considering the use of simulation gaming activities, the teacher should take into account the particular learning styles or learning preferences of the students involved.

DEVELOPING A SIMULATION GAME

If some type of simulation game appears to be an appropriate activity for specific objectives and specific students, the teacher can begin development activities leading to its use in the teaching-learning process. Development activities include investigating the possibilities of purchasing externally produced simulation games or producing a new one, and arranging for its use as a teaching-learning activity.

Depending on the teacher's time, purposes, and interest, the most reasonable approach to developing a simulation game is usually to investigate what can be currently purchased and adopted for a specific course. Regrettably, a simulation game frequently must be selected sight unseen or only on the basis of information obtained from an index or catalogue. Publishers cannot generally afford to send simulation games out on approval, as individual units can be quite costly. It should be remembered, however, that one activity can have sufficient materials for repeated plays with hundreds of students. Hence, to write for an examination copy may be akin to asking for 50 copies of one textbook. Sample kits are available at low cost for a very few simulation games; most, however, are simply too complex for this practice to be possible. It is unfortunate that the economics of publishing complicate the teacher's decision, but for the present time, until more schools have media centers or libraries that can acquire sample copies, there is no clear solution.

If a simulation game or a sample kit has been acquired, the teacher should first examine it carefully to determine its suitability for the objectives, students, classroom set-up, and specific time and resource constraints. Simulation games are seldom identified any more specifically than "for junior high and older," which means that teachers must determine whether the one received is at the right level of sophistication.

Several approaches to evaluating commercial or externally produced simulation games are available to the teacher. One generally applicable approach suggests that the following criteria be examined carefully (8):

1. Is a *central problem* presented? The problem should be clearly evident from the activity's introduction and objectives, should indicate the conceptual content of the activity, and should readily demonstrate its relationship to the real world.

2. What kind of *choices* are available to participants? The choices or alternative modes of action should allow all participants to become involved in decision making that reflects all the stated dimensions of the problem.

3. Are participants provided *different moves or activities*? All alternative courses of action should be consistent, so that major strategies selected will cause participants to make contradictory choices or moves.

4. How do the *rules* guide participant behavior? The rules of the activity should avoid distortion, which occurs when a rule overemphasizes a losing strategy, e.g., makes it easy to make a mistake but very difficult to correct it. Rules should also directly relate to the activity's problem; a winning strategy following the rules should maximize a successful resolution of the problem situation, while a losing strategy should minimize it.

5. How is the activity *organized*? All participants should be included in the essential choices and major activities; none should be assigned "observer" roles. The specific activities of the simulation game should be well conceived, consistent, and representative of real-world activities.

6. How are *summary activities* employed? A summary or debriefing period is essential to the ultimate effectiveness of the activity as a learning experience. It should bring together the basic concepts and relationships of the activity as well as suggest ways in which participants can apply what they learned.

In evaluating an externally produced simulation game, the teacher should also consider several practical characteristics (3). For example, how readily available is the activity, and what are the costs involved? Does it require a large, flexible space? Is there a high level of noise generated by participants engaged in the activity? How many players can play at once? How much preparation prior to play does the simulation game require, and how long on the average does it take to play? If the answers to these questions coincide with the teacher's purposes and resources, the activity is likely to be an effective learning experience.

If externally produced materials are inappropriate or unavailable, teachers might consider designing and constructing their own. Courses, workshops, or conferences on simulation games are the most helpful resources available to an interested teacher. These can be supplemented by readily available published materials that detail the design and construction of simulation games (see especially Maidment and Bronstein in the Unit 2 bibliography). The teacher following any one of several approaches will, in general, establish activity objectives, develop a working model and requisite materials, and try out the activity with a pilot group of students.

After selecting the type of simulation game that best fits the specific learning objectives of a course, the teacher formulates the objectives of the activity itself and decides on pertinent content to include by reviewing both personal experiences and the professional literature. Personal experience, particularly in a clinical setting, can provide the basic framework for many problem-solving activities. Drawing on personal experience can be particularly helpful for the teacher developing simulation games for the first time, for it ensures the teacher's familiarity with the problem situation, with the alternatives that were considered, and with the solution finally chosen.

Literature in the field can also provide suggestions for specific content or approaches to content for fact- or information-oriented activities. The literature review, conducted in the same fashion as it would be in preparing for a lecture or research project, can be quite helpful for such things as assigning weights or points to specific content; enumerating rules, instructions, or procedures; or developing criteria for evaluating participants' performance.

The next general step entails constructing a working model of the simulation game. A working model comprises the roles, resources, interactions, and goals that participants will encounter within the context of the simulated situation. It provides the substance for the simulation game and should be related directly to the problem and objectives already stated.

A flow chart is a useful vehicle for outlining the working model. The objectives, rationale, description of participants, needed materials, and any corresponding explanations are placed on the left side of the chart; basic rules, activities (such as assignment of roles, card plays, participant moves, etc.), and the end result or goal of the simulation game are placed on the right. These elements are generally then developed in the sequence indicated in Figure 6.1. Once the basic elements have been identified and sketched out, the teacher-designer works back and forth across both sides of the chart, refining objectives, structure, rules, and activities to ensure that each is appropriate and properly related to the others. The addition of an unanticipated but necessary activity, for example, may require the recomposition of assigned groups, which in turn may cause one or more rules to be altered.

At least one tryout, if not several, should be mandatory, particularly for the novice designer. Even the simplest simulation game is likely to have some logistical or material flaw that has gone unnoticed during the design and construction process. Tryouts not only serve as a quality control, they also allow teachers and students to develop a comfortable familiarity with the simulation-game activity.

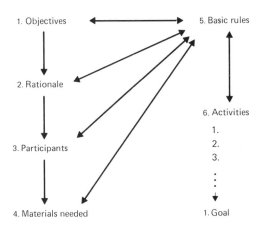

Fig. 6.1
Outline for sample simulation game flowchart.

DECIDING ON THE USE OF SIMULATION GAMES

The development of a simulation game includes deciding on the best method for using it as a teaching-learning activity. A number of authors have vividly described step-by-step methods of implementation, thus making it tempting for the teacher to "lift" selected activities in total from these sources and take them into the classroom exactly as written. Following such a procedure, however, denies the importance of participant characteristics and the need for adjusting the activity to fit a teacher's purposes, situation, and resources. Teachers should familiarize themselves with the suggested methods, but should consider them only as examples of what might be done.

On a general level, thoroughness in the preparation of a simulation game will bolster a teacher's confidence in using the activity and help ensure that a good pace will be maintained throughout its administration. The teacher's expressed confidence and enthusiasm will encourage similar reactions by students.

On a specific level, consideration of the timing of the activity is important for decisions concerning its use. There are three aspects involved in timing: choice of the time to introduce the exercise in the course or unit; choice of the time during the class period when the activity should be implemented; and choice of the time to clarify the central comments, principles, or focus of the activity.

Once a repertoire of activities has been created, particular simulation games can be held in reserve until the right time for each occurs in the schedule of the course. The "right time," for example, can be dictated by the sequence of the course's or unit's learning objectives. A nonsimulation game intended to assist students achieve minimal competence objectives may be scheduled as the primary teaching-learning activity associated with those objectives. Or, it may be scheduled to follow other activities to reinforce, sum up, or tie together information or concepts. The "right time" might also be dictated by the constraints of time or number of students. A large-system simulation game, for example, may have to be scheduled during discussion sessions and be handled by discussion leaders in a course with a lecture enrollment of 130 students.

The choice of the time during a class period when the activity should be implemented usually depends on the length of the activity. Most activities, with follow-up discussion or debriefing sessions, require a full class session. Those that need less time to complete can be scheduled as would any other teaching-learning activity, with the provision that sufficient time be allowed for the follow-up session. If a simulation game is being used for the first time, it is usually best to begin it as soon as possible in the class period. Because of various unknowns, class time may run out before the new activity is completed. If this happens, it is generally better to stop the activity, even though not completed, rather than continue hurriedly or skip important points. In such instances students generally look forward to the next class with special anticipation. Thus, the flexible teacher can turn what could have been a missed opportunity into an extended, effective learning experience, at the same time making mental notes to modify the activity the next time it is used.

The choice of time to clarify central comments, principles, or focus depends on the nature and the purpose of the exercises. Clarifications, reiterations, or reinforcements can be given on a regular basis during the activity, an approach that might be appropriate when assisting students through a nonsimulation game being used as a remedial exercise. A debriefing or discussion session approach, scheduled once at the end of an exercise, is most appropriate when students are to find their own way through decision-making or problem-solving activities.

Simulation games must be appropriate for particular students' personalities, values, general and specialized knowledge, experiences, and knowledge of one another. Some students have great difficulty role playing, sometimes to the point of experiencing extreme anxiety. To impose an elaborate or sensitive role-playing situation on such students may create severe problems. In some classes, topics involving subjects such as premarital sex, homosexuality, and venereal disease still cannot be openly discussed. Exercises on self-disclosure, stereotyping, or ranking of one's peers may be affected either by familiarity with other participants or the lack of it. All of these factors need to be considered when deciding on the methods for using a simulation game in the teaching-learning process.

The teacher's role also affects the use of the simulation game. An essential aspect is flexibility. Being prepared for fluctuations in group size caused by absences, for example, is an important characteristic of the flexible teacher. If a topic for discussion does not generate much response, it might be well to try another topic. If students are floundering in an activity, they should be assisted, so that the goal or the approach of the problem can be reestablished.

Conversely, it may happen that a teacher has intended to conclude an exercise just as students begin to get into the spirit of it. Instead of maintaining the schedule, it may be more helpful to the students for the teacher to continue a bit longer than planned. Since students are asked to demonstrate flexibility in carrying out these activities, the teacher should also display this characteristic in setting up, administering, and evaluating them.

Finally, one of the teacher's most important role functions is that of process observer. Significant events often occur during simulations without participants being aware of them; the alert teacher can provide valuable input to the players during debriefing and postactivity discussions. The role of process observer is therefore anticipated and prepared for as part of the general design activities, for it requires intimate knowledge of the components of the simulation game, the potential routes to be taken to achieve its goal, and the real-world system or institution it simulates.

REFERENCES

1. ABT, CLARK C. *Serious Games.* New York: Viking, 1970.
2. BRUNER, JEROME S. *Toward a Theory of Instruction.* Cambridge, Mass.: Harvard University Press, 1966.
3. CLARK, C. "Simulation Gaming: A New Teaching Strategy in Nursing Education." *Nurse Educator* 1 (1976): 4–9.

4. COLEMAN, JAMES S. et al. "The Hopkins Games Program: Conclusions from Seven Years of Research." *Educational Research* 2 (1973): 3–7.

5. DEARTH, SUSAN, AND LEON MCKENZIE. "Synoptics: A Simulation Game for Health Professional Students." *Journal of Continuing Education in Nursing* 6 (1975).

6. DENIKE, LEE. "An Exploratory Study of the Relationship of Educational Cognitive Style to Learning from Simulation Games." *Simulation and Games* 1 (1976): 65–74.

7. FORWARD, JOHN et al. "Teacher Control Strategies and Choice of Educational Objectives Among College Students." *Journal of Educational Psychology* 67 (1975): 757–763.

8. GILLESPIE, JUDITH A. "Analyzing and Evaluating Classroom Games." *Social Education* 36 (1972): 33–42.

9. HEGARTY, W. HARVEY. "Changes in Student Attitudes as a Result of Participating in a Simulated Game." *Journal of Educational Psychology* 67 (1975): 136–140.

10. LOWE, JEAN. "Games and Simulations in Nurse Education." *Nursing Mirror* 141 (1975): 68–69.

11. MCGUIRE, CHRISTINE. "Simulation Technique in the Teaching and Testing of Problem-Solving Skills." *Journal of Research in Science Teaching* 13 (1976): 89–100.

12. MAIDMENT, ROBERT, AND RUSSELL H. BRONSTEIN. *Simulation Games.* Columbus, Ohio: Merrill, 1973.

13. STERNBLER, WILLIAM A. "Cognitive Effects of a Programmed Simulation." *Simulation and Games* 6 (1975): 392–403.

14. STOLL, CLARICE C. "Games Students Play." *Media and Methods* 7 (1970): 37–40.

15. TWELKER, PAUL A., AND K. LAYDEN. "A Basic Reference Shelf on Simulation and Gaming." In David Zukerman and Robert Horn, eds., *The Guide to Simulation Games for Education and Training.* Cambridge, Mass.: Information Resources, Inc. 1970.

16. WEAVER, RICHARD L. "The Use of Exercises and Games." *The Speech Teacher* 23 (1974): 302–311.

7
LEARNING
PACKAGES

The teacher's development efforts result in the acquisition or production of resource materials intended to support the teaching-learning activities planned for a course or unit. When combined with other elements, such as learning objectives, a class schedule, and learning activities, they form the basic substance of the teaching-learning process. The teacher's last development activity is to organize all these elements for student use.

Two basic organizational approaches, the syllabus and the learning package, are available. Both lend themselves to several variations, permitting teachers to be flexible in the way they organize activities and materials and present them to students. The specific organizational approach taken will be based on the teacher's experience, view of students, and plans for managing the course.

A *syllabus* is an organizational tool that facilitates student learning by providing a road map to the course or unit. It presents the overall description and goals of the course, as well as the schedule of course activities, such as clinical experiences or field trips. In addition, it describes course evaluation policies and attendance requirements, and can include student self-assessment tests, individual study guides, and course and instructor evaluation forms.

A syllabus presents basic, essential information to students about the content and the conduct of a course. It is equally appropriate to a didactic-based course, to one employing the seminar-discussion format, and to one offering one or more independent-study options. It should therefore be an integral part of a teacher's first transactions with students, for even the simplest syllabus conveys a sense of planning and organization and can be used by students to guide their own approaches to the course and its activities.

A *learning package* is an organizational strategy that brings together learning activities, resource materials, and other elements into self-contained units, so that specific concepts, attitudes, or skills can be studied independently. The purpose of a package is to individualize discrete parts of the teaching-learning process by providing students with several alternative approaches to the same objectives. Students with different learning styles or preferences can therefore work toward specific objectives on an independent, self-directed basis.

A special form of the learning package, the *adjunct program*, was discussed in Chapter 5; it is developed according to the principles underlying programmed instruction. It parallels the learning package in that it brings together materials and activities to provide an independent-study option for students. It differs from the learning package in that it also organizes content. Because content is programmed, the students' approach to it is prearranged by the teacher, thus eliminating the element of self-direction (2).

Learning packages and adjunct programs necessitate the ready availability of a variety of resources and activities which students can choose from to achieve specific objectives. They also require a commitment by the teacher to provide independent-study opportunities for students. Either organizing strategy can be easily developed by the teacher with some experience, one who has taught a course or unit at least once and has acquired or produced appropriate materials and resources.

THE SYLLABUS

The basic organizational tool for bringing together the elements of a course is the syllabus. It can be quite simple in form, comprised of no more than a listing of course objectives, class schedule, and activities; or it can be quite complex, approaching the learning package in content and sophistication. The form the syllabus takes depends on the teacher's experience with the course or unit; a new teacher should try to describe at least the basic elements of the course, while seasoned teachers should be as comprehensive in their syllabus construction as resources and materials permit.

Several elements combine to form a syllabus. They can be modified as necessary to fit the teacher's purpose and the objectives of a particular course or unit.

Introductory information is included to provide an immediate overview of the course. This information includes the course title and number, overall goals, a brief description of content and the way it will be conducted, and a listing of teaching faculty and their office or conference hours.

A *listing of resources* indicates to students the type of materials that will be used in the course. The listing includes texts, journals, common reference materials, media, equipment, or any other materials students must purchase, rent, or obtain from the teacher, such as laboratory coats or aprons. Resources should be identified as required, recommended, or supplemental, and their locations given if they are to be found outside the classroom, e.g., in a learning resource center.

A *description of evaluation procedures and policies* completes the overview of the course or unit. The procedures for assessing student learning are indicated, as are the policies to be followed for assigning grades or arriving at pass-fail decisions. If a pretest and self-assessments are to be used, they can be included in the syllabus, as can the course and instructor-evaluation form.

The *format* of the course, its content and structure, comprises the major part of the syllabus. In describing the format, the teacher uses the class or activity schedule as a basic framework and fills it in with specific learning objectives and their associated learning activities and resource materials. Both developmental and minimal competence objectives could be listed down one side of a page, for example, in the sequence students will confront them in the course. Opposite the objectives would be the corresponding learning activities and/or materials students could use to work toward specific objectives.

The syllabus provides a convenient, efficient, and permanent guide for students as they progress through a course or unit. It can also be, for the teacher, a convenient, efficient, and permanent means of communicating with students.

LEARNING PACKAGES

The teacher is probably the most flexible resource available to individual students in a course. It is possible for the teacher to speed up a presentation, discussion, or demonstration; slow one down; encourage critical thinking in an area; or set limits on a topic or discussion that is beyond the scope of specific objectives. To be such a flexible resource and to provide a type of individualized instruction, the teacher must be able to actively transact with each student. Active transactions are possible when there is immediate, two-way communication between the teacher and student. Teachers charged with 130 students per course will find it virtually impossible to engage in such transactions with each student.

Learning packages help a teacher organize and manage a course with a large number of students and, at the same time, permit active transactions with individual students. By providing individualized, self-directed learning opportunities for students, learning packages allow the teacher to maximize opportunities for personal work with students who request it. In addition to allowing for more teacher-student interactions, learning packages can free up time for teachers to engage in activities that otherwise might not receive adequate attention, specifically, tutoring, clarifying issues, amplifying ideas, and encouraging and stimulating the learning of individual students. In essence, learning packages serve a double function: they give the teacher more time to facilitate growth in each student, while ensuring that the established standards of a course are maintained.

Learning packages allow a teacher to manage a course so students can proceed at their own pace, according to their individual needs and learning styles. It may be possible for students to begin their study of parts of a course at any time during the semester or rotation without having to wait for a designated "start." Learning packages encourage students to accomplish a great deal of the course independently; they are freed from having to attend lectures or other formalized activities. Such packages replace the teacher in the sense that each student decides how learning will progress, rather than having this directed by the teacher.

Since learning packages organize a variety of materials into small, self-contained units, it is possible for students at any time in a course to assess their own individual progress. Learning packages therefore can provide students, as well as the teacher, with ongoing information about student progress. Learning problems that may be expressed in students' inability to pace themselves through a course can be identified early, so the teacher and students can have time to work on them together.

The majority of students can manage their own learning if given the opportunity. Past learning experiences should be utilized to the fullest extent, so that students do not become frustrated, bored, or discouraged with teacher-directed learning. By the same token, many students come to feel inadequate, frustrated, or anxious about their learning. Learning situations controlled by others (e.g., by a teacher in a classroom) often instill in students a feeling of vulnerability, so that they may be afraid to make a mistake and eventually begin to doubt their own abilities (3). With learning packages, teachers can develop courses that give control over learning method, pace, and timing to students who desire such control.

There is no standard outline or format dictating what a learning package should contain. Teachers using learning packages should be careful to design each one as a separate entity. The package should reflect the specific objectives of the content or course unit it represents, the particular discipline involved, and the available resources. Thus, for a unit on circulatory diseases, a statement of prerequisites to the unit would be important, since it would clearly define the necessary knowledge of anatomy and physiology that must be mastered before students begin work with the package. A unit on the concept of grieving, on the other hand, might not contain any prerequisites. An adjunct program on the pharmacology of antidepressants would structure student activities and restrict students to specific materials; a learning package on the same content would provide alternative activities or materials that students could use at their discretion to achieve the unit's learning objectives. The teacher should thus avoid following a constant format or outline when developing learning packages, but rather should be flexible and adapt each package to the needs and requirements of specific objectives, content, and resources.

While there is no standard format dictating the contents of learning packages, there are several components teachers usually include when developing specific packages. These components are a statement of prerequisites; a listing of specific learning objectives; one or more assessment devices; a series of alternative learning activities; and a description of available resource materials.

Statement of Prerequisites

Prerequisite knowledge, skills, or abilities frequently are not clearly spelled out for students. A teacher may assume, for example, that if students have had a course in normal nutrition they will remember that one gram of fat has nine calories. Many students may remember this fact from a previous course, although many may not. Retention and recall of prerequisite information can directly influence the progress students can expect to make in subsequent learning experiences. Too frequently, students begin a new unit, have difficulty with some aspect of the material presented, and become frustrated and discouraged. Teachers may attribute this difficulty to the content being studied or to the students' motivation or methods of learning when, in actuality, it may be related to the teacher's incorrect assumptions about previous learning.

A general statement of prerequisites, such as, "An understanding of normal nutrition," is not helpful. A more helpful statement referring to the same area would be: "Can use the four basic food groups to plan a daily diet for a normal adolescent." Depending on the academic or ability levels of the students who will be using the learning package, it may be appropriate and helpful to the students to include resources to consult if prerequisites are missing.

Learning Objectives

Learning packages usually begin with an overview of the unit—i.e., a concise statement of the unit's purposes and its relationship to other course components or learning packages. The overview indicates to students what the unit will be about, as well as the rationale for using the learning package.

Following the overview, and providing specific direction for the students beginning the learning package, are the specific learning objectives forming the basis of the package. Both minimal and developmental competence objectives can be included, although minimal competence objectives are usually more appropriate, since they represent knowledge, skills, or behaviors students should be able to master on their own. Through transacting with the teacher and other students, either at some designated point in the package or following its use, students can approach developmental competence objectives. This type of objective would usually be included to provide students with in-depth, independent-study options.

Assessment Devices

Each learning package should contain a pretest students complete before beginning the unit's activities. The pretest is intended to help students assess their own level of competence in the specific content area of the learning package. The pretest provides the teacher with entry data on each student and gives each student feedback useful in determining the proper amount of time to spend on the unit's activities.

The pretest may be a pencil-and-paper test of the knowledge, skills, or behaviors called for by the objectives. Or, it may be a laboratory exercise, a videotape, or based on clinical or other resources. Whichever format the teacher selects, it should allow sampling of all the objectives of the unit.

If the pretests are well constructed and test-result information is available from previous groups of students, it should be possible to assemble several pretests to provide a credit-by-examination alternative for students. Thus, a student could challenge all or a part of a course easily, while the teacher is still able to maintain traditional course standards. With this type of testing students can accelerate their progress through learning packages they have mastered and spend more time on units that are difficult for them, or on an in-depth independent-study project, or on the next learning package. It may also be possible for the teacher to further personalize the course by clustering students according to their test results.

Self-assessment examinations should be included with each set of learning activities included in a learning package. Thus, students choosing any one of three different learning activities to meet specific objectives can complete the same self-assessment examination referenced to the objectives in question. The information obtained from the examinations will help uncover individual weaknesses, indicate that another activity or resource might best be used to achieve the objectives, or encourage the student to go on to another set of activities or to another learning package.

Learning Activities

The heart of a learning package is the activities it includes. From these, students choose those activities they wish to pursue to accomplish the objectives of the unit. Since students come to any course with a variety of learning styles and preferences, it is most helpful to them if teachers can provide, in learning packages, as many alternative learning activities as possible. Thus, there may be a reading assignment, an audio cassette, and a slide-tape program, all referenced directly to the same objectives. In this case, each student has the option of either reading, hearing, or hearing and seeing specific content.

Previous assessments of learner characteristics are beneficial to the teacher in selecting appropriate learning activities. The teacher considers the learning styles or preferences of students who have previously taken the course and selects at least three different learning activities for the same learning objective. For example, one of the learning activities might be especially appropriate for audiovisual-oriented students, while another might be directed at students who prefer the more active participation programmed instruction provides. The teacher should be as persistent and as creative as possible at this point in seeking out a variety of activities and determining which ones are readily available, which ones should be scheduled for preview before purchase, and which ones should be developed.

The following types of activities could be effective as alternatives available to students in a learning package:

- Reading assignments, e.g., journal articles, text sections
- Film/videotape/slide-tape program
- Laboratory assignment
- Demonstration
- Programmed instruction
- Skill practice session
- Simulation game
- Conference
- Field trip
- Field experiment
- Project

Some of these activities entail independent work on the part of students; some require teacher participation, either on a small-group or individualized basis; others permit in-depth, independent study by students electing to go beyond the basic requirements of the package. The teacher's selection of activities thus depends on the nature of the learning objectives; on the types of students expected to use the package; on the availability of materials, or on the ease with which new materials can be developed; and on the teacher's interest in and ability to schedule small-group and individualized sessions with students to complement the basic activities of the package.

After completing the selection of activities, the next step is to write a study guide. The study guide should clearly describe for the student all the parameters of the learning activities of the package. For example, if a learning package on transplantation immunology has an objective that requires students to view slides depicting the types of allograft rejection, the study guide should include the location of the slides, their call numbers on a learning resource center, or any other special directions that will be necessary to ensure a successful, efficient learning experience. An incorrect title on a slide-tape program, for example, may cost the student lost time in unproductive hunting and searching.

Oftentimes students will already have had some experience with self-directed learning using media in previous courses; for others it will be a totally new experience. If a course has a large number of media resources, it usually is helpful for students as part of their orientation to the course and to the learning packages to be shown the library or center where media is kept and to have an opportunity to learn how to operate the necessary equipment. Such an orientation can save learning time for students and repair time for the staff of the library or media center, for equipment can be broken and out of use for long periods of time if students are not familiar with its proper use.

Resource Materials

Resource materials are those that students receive with a learning package and retain for their own use. They can include such things as worksheets, study questions, case studies, interviewing or assessment tools, and sample test questions. Rather than continually developing and passing out material to students, resource materials can be coordinated with specific learning activities and included in the appropriate place in the learning package. More extensive resources, such as a copy of a paper intended to replace a lecture, a taxonomy, or a monograph series, can either be included as required experiences or referenced and suggested as optional experiences.

An additional, essential resource is the bibliography. The bibliography contains a listing of pertinent written references, as well as other types of reference materials, such as audiovisuals, pamphlets, or indices. Required reading assignments should be noted here; when entries represent duplicate materials, students should be informed they need read only one or the other. If more than one entry needs to be consulted to meet a specific objective, however, students should be so alerted. The bibliography is particularly important also for suggesting in-depth approaches to specific content areas, for encouraging further independent study, and for introducing approaches to any developmental competence objectives included in the package.

Pilot Testing

Once a learning package has been developed, the teacher should pilot test it with a small group of students. It is usually suggested that the pilot students (at least four or five) be asked to respond to three areas after they have completed the package (1). These are common problem areas, and involve clarity, student attention, and methods of instruction.

Problems of *clarity* occur when materials are included in a learning package that may be equivocal, imprecise, or not readily understandable. They may need to be rewritten, redefined, or expanded. Based on the information obtained from the pilot group, the teacher may simplify an explanation, reword instructions, or delete some materials and add new ones in their place.

Another common problem area is *student attention*. The learning package may not be able to hold student interest, arouse curiosity, or provide sufficient challenge. Students may find it boring, distracting, or overwhelming. The problems of attention identified by the pilot group may necessitate a revision of the overview or rationale of the package, an alteration of the level of difficulty of the learning activities or resources, or a change in the instructions and progression of activities comprising the package.

The last area to be assessed by the pilot group should be the *methods of instruction* employed in the package. There may be problems of presentation due to pacing, sequencing, organization, size of package, or opportunities for practice and reinforcement. The feedback obtained from the pilot group indicates to the teacher what methods of presentation need to be modified before the learning package is finalized. It may also provide direction for revising the formats or schedule of small-group or individualized encounters that involve student-teacher interactions.

After the learning package is revised, based on the information provided by the pilot group, it is ready for use by an entire class. The same three areas should be evaluated by the total group to determine if the same or different problems exist in the package.

Developing a Course Composed of Learning Packages

A teacher developing a series of related learning packages or a number of separate learning packages has the opportunity to construct a course or unit, either in whole or in part, around student use of the packages. Several configurations in course or unit construction are possible with learning packages. For instance, if there is an introductory unit now available as a learning package, followed by several self-contained packages, and a final package that summarizes the content unit or course, the following could graphically represent for the students the relationships of the packages to each other:

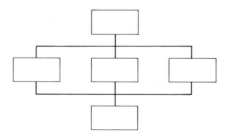

A course or unit where all the learning packages are self-contained would be represented by the following illustration. It indicates that the packages can be studied in any order:

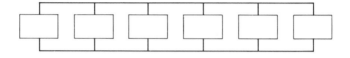

If there is a particular order in which the learning packages are to be studied, students should also be told this in advance. The following illustration represents a course or unit in which the student could modify the sequence of only some of the learning packages:

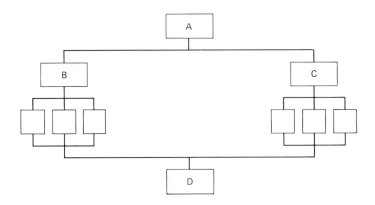

A sequence could be ABCD or ACBD, but always A and D would be first and last, respectively.

Using any of these configurations of learning packages to conduct a course or unit can benefit slow learners, fast learners, students taking the course as a requirement, as well as those simply interested in the subject content. The teacher can use learning packages to provide students with opportunities for remedial work, in-depth study of particular topics, or fully independent study. Such opportunities can be easily arranged for both large and small groups of students, providing the optimal form of self-directed study throughout a course or unit.

REFERENCES

1. JOHNSON, STUART R., AND RITA B. JOHNSON. *Developing Individualized Instruction Material.* New York: Westinghouse Learning Corporation, 1970.

2. MONAHAN, JAMES. "The Organization of Materials for Self-Directed Learning." In Jerome P. Lysaught, ed., *Instructional Technology in Medical Education.* New York: The Rochester Clearinghouse, University of Rochester, 1973, pp. 151-59.

3. PETERSON, MARGARET H., AND FRED D. STRIDER. "Student Preferences for Individualized Instruction." In Jerome P. Lysaught, ed., *Instructional Technology in Medical Education.* New York: The Rochester Clearinghouse, University of Rochester, 1973, pp. 55-65.

UNIT 2
BIBLIOGRAPHY

Instructional Media

A.V. Communication Review (quarterly), published by the Association for Educational Communications and Technology, 1201 Sixteenth St., N.W., Washington, D.C., Library of Congress No. AP A9123.

One of the major reference journals concerned with instructional media. Contains papers on theory, development, research, and practical applications related to technological processes in education. Regular features include book reviews and research abstracts.

BROWN, JAMES. W., RICHARD B. LEWIS, and FRED F. HARCLEROAD. *AV Instruction: Technology, Media, and Methods.* 5th ed. New York: McGraw-Hill, 1977.

A standard reference on the selection, production, and use of instructional media. The principles and procedures it presents are applicable to all levels of education. Will be useful to teachers unfamiliar with media alternatives who are interested in the possible uses of media in their teaching.

CURL, DAVID H., and CARLTON W. H. ERICKSON. *Fundamentals of Teaching with Audiovisual Technology.* New York: Macmillan, 1972.

A useful basic reference on the selection, use, and production of audiovisual materials.

DYER, CHARLES A. *Preparing for Computer Assisted Instruction.* Englewood Cliffs, N.J.: Educational Technology Publications, 1972.

Presents the basics of computer operations and the applications of computers to the teaching-learning process. Describes procedures for planning and developing a program, as well as procedures for in-service and programmer training.

ELLIS, ALLAN B. *The Use and Misuse of Computers in Education.* New York: McGraw-Hill, 1974.

Clear descriptions of the uses of computers in education. Contains a unit on the development of system software and an appendix that may be helpful for someone considering computer-assisted instruction for a course, department, or institution.

KEMP, JERROLD E. *Planning and Producing Audiovisual Materials.* 3d ed. New York: Crowell, 1975.

A good reference in the selection and use of instructional materials. Discusses selection and use of various types of media in terms of their appropriateness to the teaching-learning process.

LANGE, PHIL C., ed. *Programmed Instruction.* Sixty-sixth Yearbook of the National Society for the Study of Education. Part II. Chicago, 1976.

Presents a variety of papers describing theoretical and practical approaches to programmed instruction. A basic reference on the principles and applications of programmed instruction.

MINOR, ED, and HARVEY R. FRYE. *Techniques for Producing Visual Instructional Material.* New York: McGraw-Hill, 1977.

A comprehensive resource on the production of a variety of types of visual materials and on a variety of techniques from which the teacher can choose to produce visuals. Although a technical book, its step-by-step procedures should be understandable to the nontechnician teacher.

TEACHEY, WILLIAM G., and JOSEPH B. CARTER. *Learning Laboratories.* Englewood Cliffs, N.J.: Educational Technology Publications, 1971.

Describes the development and uses of learning laboratories; topics range from requirements for physical facilities to the role of the laboratory coordinator. Appendices contain information about evaluation materials as well as vendors and autoinstructional equipment.

WIMAN, RAYMOND V., and WESLEY C. MEIERHENRY, eds. *Educational Media, Theory into Practice.* Columbus, Ohio: Merrill, 1969.

A collection of papers describing several theoretical and practical approaches to instructional media. Useful as a reference on the issues involved in selecting and using media.

Simulation Games

ABT, CLARK C. *Serious Games.* New York: Viking, 1970.

A comprehensive treatment of games as teaching-learning strategies. Discusses their principles, procedures, implications, and applications. A basic reference.

ADAMS, DENNIS M. *Simulation Games: An Approach to Learning.* Worthington, Ohio: Charles A. Jones, 1973.

A straightforward discussion of the design and use of simulations. Includes a sampling of commercially prepared and teacher-made simulation games, many of which could form the bases for adaptation to other classroom situations or the development of new simulation-game activities.

BOOCOCK, SARANE S., and E. O. SCHILD, eds. *Simulation Games in Learning.* Beverly Hills, Ca.: Sage, 1968.

A collection of papers describing the development of simulation games as legitimate teaching-learning strategies.

MAIDMENT, ROBERT, and RUSSELL H. BRONSTEIN. *Simulation Games—Design and Implementation.* Columbus, Ohio: Merrill, 1973.

A brief and concise text, yet one of the most useful and available on simulation games. Presents a framework for the systematic design and use of simulation games, leading the reader through a step-by-step development process.

Simulation and Games (quarterly), published by Sage Publications, Beverly Hills, California, Library of Congress No. S S14 AN2.

An international journal intended to provide a forum for theoretical, empirical, and practical application papers related to man, man-machine, and machine simulations of social processes. Includes book reviews, simulation reviews, and listings of newly available simulations. A basic resource for teachers interested in developing expertise in the development, use, and evaluation of simulation games.

TANSEY, P. J. *Educational Aspects of Simulation.* London, England: McGraw-Hill, 1971.

Papers on a variety of topics concerned with the development and use of games, simulations, nonsimulation games and simulation games. Discussions include both practical applications and the results of research conducted at various educational levels in several countries.

ZUCKERMAN, DAVID, and ROBERT E. HORN. *The Guide to Simulations/Games for Education and Training.* Lexington, Mass.: Information Resources, Inc., 1973.

A collection of papers and reports in the development, use, and evaluation of simulations and games. A basic reference for the new teacher and the teacher experienced in designing and using simulation/games.

Learning Packages

JOHNSON, STUART R., and RITA B. JOHNSON. *Developing Individualized Instructional Material.* Palo Alto, Ca.: Westinghouse Learning Press, 1971.

A small, concise book; the principles of individualizing instructional material are applicable to several areas of interest, including learning packages.

KAPFER, PHILIP G., and MIRIAM B. KAPFER, eds. *Learning Packages in American Education.* Englewood Cliffs, N.J.: Educational Technology Publications, 1972.

Directed primarily at general education. Includes discussions concerning instructional module design, learning activities, an auto-tutorial system incorporating minicourses, and classroom management of learning packages. Discussions can easily be applied to teaching in the health sciences.

UNIT 3
THE MANAGEMENT PROCESS

Teachers' planning and development activities are directed at creating opportunities for entering into transactions with students. Management activities bring together teachers and students to work toward the goals of a specific course or unit of study.

The strategies chosen to manage teaching-learning transactions may be traditional, such as lectures or structured laboratory experiences, or nontraditional, such as learning packages or contingency contracting. In following a systematic approach to teaching, teachers select those management strategies that reflect their purposes, resources, and the needs and interests of their students.

Teachers' selections of management strategies may also reflect their familiarity with specific strategies. New teachers frequently utilize traditional approaches when beginning their teaching activities, since their own educational preparation was conducted along traditional lines. More experienced teachers may feel comfortable in expanding their repertoire to include nontraditional approaches. Depending on the teacher's personal approach, both traditional and nontraditional strategies can provide students the opportunity to participate actively in the management of the teaching-learning process and can encourage them to assume greater responsibility for their own learning.

The chapters of this unit focus on the management aspects of teaching. Several traditional and nontraditional strategies teachers can use in the teaching-learning process are examined. Chapter 8 describes the traditional teaching strategies: lecture, discussion, clinical teaching, and laboratory teaching. In Chapter 9, the range of personalized instruction, from learning packages to contingency contracting to individual tutoring, is explored. A framework for group life and strategies for approaching each phase of group life are presented in Chapter 10.

8

TRADITIONAL
TEACHING
STRATEGIES

Approaches to traditional teaching strategies in the health sciences, i.e., lecture, discussion, laboratory or clinical teaching, have been influenced to a large extent by the traditional environmental constraints imposed on the teaching-learning process: institutional time schedules, space and room allocations, and classes composed of large numbers of students. Such constraints, when coupled with an emphasis on efficient preparation of practitioners, have caused these teaching strategies to become somewhat uniform and predictable. Further, because most health science teachers are thrust into teaching situations with little or no preparation or formal educational experience, the tendency to "teach as taught" predominates. This not only perpetuates uniform, predictable teaching practices, of varying quality, it also frequently causes mismatches between personal talents or abilities and specific teaching strategies.

Traditional teaching strategies can be effective means for helping students to achieve learning objectives. Any inadequacies or inefficiencies can generally be traced to specific teacher deficiencies, rather than to the strategies themselves. An understanding of and an ability to use traditional strategies effectively is an important first step in developing one's role as a teacher and in establishing the necessary background for selecting and using alternate strategies more closely matched to one's special talents and abilities.

LECTURE

The most widely used and frequently abused traditional teaching strategy is the lecture. It has been the predominant approach to teaching in higher education for centuries; in the health sciences, the lecture has its roots in medieval medical education.

The traditional purpose of the lecture has long been the transmission of knowledge. However, the lecture can be much more: it can be the means for bringing together ideas, concepts, and principles from diverse sources; for presenting both general and specific approaches to problem solving; and for encouraging students to apply previously acquired knowledge to new situations, to synthesize information based on research and opinions from diverse sources, and to develop the ability to question and evaluate, an ability they will need as life-long learners. By formulating the lecture according to one of these general purposes, the teacher can assist students in their pursuit of both mimimal and developmental competence objectives.

Teachers and students experience difficulty, frustration, and apathy with the lecture primarily because the strategy is still often used to transmit information. The failure to use alternate strategies and a variety of teaching-learning resources to transmit information places this burden on the lecture alone. And, since the lecture is the main vehicle for interaction between teacher and students, this interaction in turn is reduced to the teacher's explication of factual subject content related to minimal competence objectives. Such a teaching-learning system is largely inefficient and ineffective.

Because reading and speaking rates differ, even the slowest reader should be able to obtain more factual information by reading than by listening to a lecture, given the same amount of time for each activity. In fact, when well selected and well structured, printed materials alone can be more efficient and just as effective in enabling students to assimilate and recall information (5). Similarly, programmed instructional materials can require half the time commitment of students that lectures require and yet result in better achievement of minimal competence objectives (12). Simulation exercises and a variety of audiovisual materials can also be more effective and efficient than the lecture in assisting students to attain learning objectives (23); when used alone or in combination, these strategies can contribute to students' achievement of cognitive, affective, and skill objectives.

A variety of teaching-learning strategies and resources can replace the lecture for general informational purposes. What these alternative strategies and resources cannot always do effectively, however, is provide a live, personal means for challenging, sensitizing, stimulating, or motivating students in their pursuit of learning objectives (26). Only the teacher can do this. Therefore, the teacher should take care that this unique resource be used to the advantage of students. It can be used to their advantage in a lecture situation if the teacher views the lecture as a means of achieving purposes other than information transmission, structures the lecture following several general principles, and emphasizes positive personal attributes in its delivery.

The general teaching-learning *purposes* the lecture can serve have been mentioned previously, i.e., synthesizing, presenting approaches to problem solving, and encouraging students to develop a variety of abilities. These purposes deviate from the traditional transmission of information and represent one way in which teachers can transact with students, albeit on a large-group basis. In planning a course or unit, teachers should therefore anticipate acquiring or developing resources students can use individually or in groups to confront basic subject content. Lectures can then be planned and scheduled to provide, on one level, a unifying thread for the content of the course or unit and, on another level, the means for stimulating students' problem solving. In a unit on nutrition, for example, students may be given the opportunity to achieve minimal competence objectives dealing with the composition of protein, carbohydrates, fat, minerals, vitamins, and water by using programmed materials or slide-tape programs. The subsequent lecture might then relate nutrient deficiencies and excesses to the assessment, treatment, and prevention of specific health problems. The problem-solving approach to lectures should be especially important to teachers who are responsible for a large group of students and who, because of institutional scheduling procedures, have little opportunity for transacting with small groups of students.

In planning the *structure* of a lecture teachers must be aware of the "spurt-sag-spurt" phenomenon that is common to any teacher and group of students engaged in lecture as a teaching-learning activity (13). The first five or more minutes of a fifty-minute lecture, for example, are characterized by high efficiency on the part of both teachers and students, an initial "spurt" of high output or performance. This warm-up period is followed by a middle sag period, in which student and lecturer efficiency declines, reaching its lowest point after about 40 minutes. Both teachers and students then experience a second spurt of efficiency which moves them toward their initial level of performance. Neither reaches that level, however, with teacher performance frequently improving less than student performance.

A variety of factors contribute to the spurt-sag-spurt pattern, among them the relative difficulty of subject content, the relationship between teacher and students, the time of day of the lecture, and the physical environment of the lecture hall. These factors, alone or in combination, can result in fatigue or boredom on the part of students; the extent to which students are tired or bored will have a direct effect on their decline in efficiency during the middle part of the lecture. To reduce this decline, teachers should plan lectures that are diversified by a variety of audiovisual materials, pauses in delivery, changes of pace, and intervals for clarification of ideas, questions and answers, or problem solving (13). Such diversity is important to the success of the lecture and should be accompanied by a sensitivity to the collective needs of the students. Diversity of technique and sensitivity to student needs are elements that are specific to each teacher and each lecture; time, patience, and practice are required to achieve the right combination in structuring particular lectures.

Several general principles can be followed in structuring a lecture. When planning for a lecture, the teacher first engages in a self-questioning process intended to identify the key points of the lecture (8). By reexamining the resources made available to students to approach specific subject content and learning objectives, the teacher should answer such questions as: How can this lecture bring together information and ideas students should already possess to encourage problem solving? If students were to learn only one thing from this lecture, what would it be? Answers to these questions help to identify the key points of the lecture and its logical sections.

When key points have been identified, the lecture can be organized in several logical sections or units, each designed to comprise not more than ten or fifteen minutes of lecture time (10). Nonstop discourse generally strains students' capacity for concentrated attention, causes continuity of thought to be lost, and significantly decreases performance efficiency in the "sag" portion of the lecture. Breaks between lecture sections, which need not be long, can consist of brief discussions with students, question-and-answer sessions, or a problem exercise. These breaks allow students to participate verbally in lectures.

A lecture must stimulate students intellectually and make them active participants in it (8). Active participation here refers to student involvement in the thought processes of the lecture. This participation can be encouraged by distributing an outline of the lecture at the beginning; opening the lecture with a statement of its key points; including opportunities for clarification at designated intervals; presenting problems that require independent, postlecture effort for solution; asking test-type questions periodically to reinforce material and stimulate discussion; and relating theory to practical applications where appropriate. Audiovisual materials, such as slides, videotapes, or overhead transparencies, can be effective supplementary devices for encouraging intellectual participation by students, as well as for minimizing student fatigue and boredom.

Active participation by students can also be encouraged if the teacher outlines the lecture and includes salient notes within the outline, but does not write the lecture out to be read verbatim. A lecture read in its entirety usually serves to increase the probability that the middle "sag" of the lecture will reach a low limit of inefficiency. The teacher concerned with time usage in the lecture should note in the margins of the lecture outline the amount of time to be spent on each section of the lecture.

Personal attributes of teachers contribute greatly to the overall effectiveness of their lectures. Vocal qualities such as pitch, projection, enunciation, modulation, and rate of delivery; gestures or other uses of physical self to emphasize, persuade, or motivate; and ability to develop rapport with students can have an effect on student learning (27). Few teachers are well equipped and competent in each of these areas when they begin teaching; they attain proficiency through interest in self-improvement and practice. Perhaps the best way to develop these attributes is to seek help from an experienced teacher or educational consultant, someone who is well versed in the construction and delivery of lectures and in public-speaking techniques. The teacher and colleague should first identify the teacher's strengths and weaknesses, perhaps through microteaching; decide on an approach to lecturing that emphasizes the teacher's current strengths; and agree on a practice schedule for dealing with weaknesses and trying out new lecture techniques as a course or unit progresses.

SMALL-GROUP DISCUSSION

A small-group discussion is a purposeful, systematic, oral exchange of ideas by a group of individuals who share in the leadership of the group (20). Teacher and students interact through discussion to establish satisfactory generalizations, conclusions, or solutions. At the same time, the small-group setting promotes positive interpersonal relationships among the members of the group (6). This teaching strategy, which encourages a cognitive approach to teaching and learning, can be the primary strategy used in a course or unit, as in an advanced course developed around a series of seminars. It can also be used to supplement large-group activities, as in discussion sections scheduled for students enrolled in a lecture-oriented course.

To be effective in contributing to student learning, the discussion must be *purposeful;* it must have a goal or goals that are clearly identified, understood, and accepted by the group. Because the discussion can be a highly effective means for approaching developmental competence objectives, it might best be developed around one central, multifaceted problem or a small group of related problems. In this way the statement of the problem situation, made available to students in advance of the discussion session, serves not only to bring together relevant minimal competence objectives and related materials before the discussion, but also to focus students' thinking as the actual discussion takes place.

Problem solving associated with developmental competence objectives is necessarily directed at multifaceted problems, those with a variety of parts and the potential for multiple solutions. This characteristic is inherent in the nature of such objectives. The use of discussion is therefore an appropriate teaching-learning strategy for approaching developmental competence objectives, for students can accomplish more working in small groups than by acting individually (2). Solutions to multifaceted problems require the contributions of students with diverse talents, backgrounds, points of view, and academic abilities, a diversity that usually can be arranged for in assigning seminar or discussion groups. Students of above-average, average, and below-average ability have specific contributions to make to the problem-solving process; each one can benefit in one way or another from the others' contributions.

A good discussion directed at developmental competence objectives is *systematic;* it follows a logical plan, rather than the random flow that is characteristic of casual conversation. A plan for the discussion, developed after the problem or topic has been established, can include an outline, time schedule, participant duties, and required information or materials (20).

An outline or some orderly sequence of activities should provide the framework for the discussion. The framework might consist of a series of questions to be posed to members of the group at specific intervals. The questions would reflect the development of the problem from its definition to its potential solutions. It might also consist of a detailed outline of specific information, facts, or opinions that constitute the elements of the problem and are requisite to its solution. The framework chosen should be used to guide the discussion, not force it to abide by an inflexible agenda.

A time schedule is a further means of guiding the discussion from beginning to end. By knowing the approximate amount of time to be spent on each part of the intended discussion, the teacher can gauge the progression of the discussion session. While diversions, digressions, or concentrated exchanges on specific points can be quite fruitful in moving the group toward solution of the problem, they can also be detrimental to realizing the purposes of the discussion if permitted to continue beyond a reasonable amount of time. The teacher as subject-content expert and consultant to the group thus has a responsibility to allocate time, in a general fashion, to the various segments of the discussion and to share this allocation with students at the outset of the discussion session.

Participant duties are identified and agreed on before a discussion begins. These duties will vary, depending on the level of the students, the purpose of the discussion, and the nature of the problem to be investigated. Students might be requested initially to respond to a series of questions from the teacher and then to use their answers as the bases for their participation in the discussion. Or, they might be assigned or asked to choose roles to play in the discussion; this would necessitate advance preparation to ensure that role consistency is maintained during the actual discussion. Various parts of the problem situation might also be distributed among participants, so that each person can become familiar with a particular aspect of the problem and assume responsibility for moderating subsequent discussion on that topic. Further, for every type of duty given student participants, a corresponding duty must be assumed by the teacher, from director, to facilitator, to interested observer (14).

The provision of required information or materials also contributes to the systematic character of a discussion. Both teacher and students must not only know the problem to be addressed, they must also be as familiar as possible with the facts, opinions, and related information that have a bearing on the various aspects of the problem. Similarly, any equipment, references, audio-visual aids, or other materials used to facilitate the discussion must be provided and made readily available to all members of the discussion group.

Discussions are conducted to encourage the *oral exchange of ideas* among participants. Because the ultimate effectiveness of the discussion as a teaching-learning strategy is dependent on the nature of this exchange, the teacher's planning must include provisions for facilitating the exchange. Merely gathering students together in a classroom and presenting them with a problem will not ensure that reasoned discussion leading to resolution of the problem will take place. Along with the purpose and logical plan, several factors relating to the physical environment of the discussion can affect its nature and its outcome, among them lighting, ventilation, acoustics, and seating arrangement. Of these, the teacher has the greatest control over seating arrangement, which perhaps more than the other physical factors will affect the progress of the discussion.

The most trying place to conduct a small-group discussion is in a lecture hall where seats are fastened to risers. While some form of communication can take place here among discussion-group members, such an arrangement is more than likely to restrict severely participation by all members and reduce the likelihood of group problem solving (22). For effective communication to take place, all discussion participants must be able to face each other and easily see and hear one another. Using a conference table or arranging movable chairs in the shape of a horseshoe or circle will promote the exchange of ideas and the building of mutual trust among participants (8).

The seating arrangement selected can significantly affect the communication patterns of the discussion group. When the teacher faces all participants, as in a lecture situation, a centralized communication pattern in which the teacher dominates the flow of the discussion is likely to occur. This arrangement is usually less satisfactory and less productive for group members than a decentralized discussion pattern, achieved when group members are seated in a face-to-face arrangement. A decentralized pattern permits the free flow of information and efficient and accurate problem solving (3). While such a pattern initially takes longer for participants to adjust to and find manageable, it eventually is more effective than centralized communication.

The composition of the *group of individuals* engaging in discussion affects both the process and the product of the discussion. Although a discussion can take place satisfactorily with from two to twenty students (4), the optimum number of students in a discovery-oriented, problem-solving discussion is five (7). A group size of less than five decreases the possibility of diversity, while a greater size limits the possibility of all members participating actively. Further, an odd-numbered group ensures that deadlocks in deliberation, voting, and decision making can be avoided—a group of five, for example, may split 3 to 2 on specific issues, but still continue its work toward resolution of the problem at hand.

Seating arrangements and group size contribute significantly to the oral exchange among group members. While participation by all members is highly desirable and is the objective guiding the development of small-group discussion, teachers should not be concerned if one or more students choose to assume quiet observer roles during parts of a discussion. That all students do not participate during a given time period does not mean they are not learning or are dissatisfied with the group process (19). On the contrary, students can be actively involved in listening and thinking without making continued oral contributions to the discussion.

The individuals engaging in a discussion must be able to *share in the leadership of the group*. Leadership can be shared if the teacher relinquishes the traditional position of authority and becomes a member of the group, albeit a member with a more sophisticated background and a firmer grasp of the subject content at hand. The teacher can initially act as leader to begin the group's discussion process and then turn over leadership either by appointing a student leader, encouraging students to elect leaders on a rotating basis, assigning leadership roles to accompany specific content or aspects of the discussion, or allowing leaders to emerge naturally from the general membership of the group. The type of shared leadership most appropriate for specific groups is dependent on the nature of the group members (6). The teacher's ability to assess student needs and interests and to recognize the character of each group, an ability developed through working with groups, can be helpful in determining the type of leadership needed in specific situations.

CLINICAL TEACHING

Clinical teaching-learning experiences afford students opportunities to learn how to interact with people seeking health care, with people providing it, and with the organization in which these two meet. The purpose of clinical experiences is to assist students in gaining mastery of the methods needed to deal effectively with these interactions, as well as mastery of the knowledge, insight, and skills required to function capably as health-care professionals.

The learning climate established by the teacher should capitalize on the freedom and independence that can be afforded students. At the same time, the teacher must recognize the need to be available for help, assistance, or consultation. Teachers should encourage students' curiosity, provide support when students question current ideas and practice, and give them ample opportunity to test and evaluate new ideas.

It is not unusual for students to be anxious in clinical environments. The fear of making a fatal mistake or the anxiety associated with an unfamiliar situation may be overwhelming. Frustration generated by the reality of providing care in an institution can also become acute. Students have their own standards by which they measure their clinical effectiveness. If these self-imposed standards are higher than those expected by the teacher, the student may experience frustration and despair. Most often, though, students are challenged, eager, and involved in their clinical learning experiences and this enthusiasm can be enhanced by the teacher.

The teacher needs to accept first that students will not and should not become rubber-stamped practitioners. Clinical situations provide students with the opportunity to individualize their goals and their approaches to health care according to their personal styles and basic beliefs. While most teachers are comfortable in encouraging a wide variety of student clinical behaviors, certain assumptions about students can help the teacher participate effectively in clinical learning (21).

The first assumption is that all students are potentially capable of functioning satisfactorily in the clinical area. Acceptance of this assumption allows the teacher to trust students with independence and responsibility as they interact with patients. A second assumption is that, at any given moment, students operate according to their best judgment. Thus, if a student makes a mistake or is functioning at a low level, while this may be unacceptable or even dangerous, it is the best level at which the student can currently function—he or she is not intentionally behaving in a dangerous way. Teachers also need to assume that students are genuinely interested in the profession and will both seek out and accept help if the teacher has provided an environment in which this is acceptable behavior.

Clinical teaching, then, is helping the student to self-discovery. The teacher encourages this learning by developing a sense of when to offer assistance and guidance and when to allow students to manage on their own.

Planning and Selecting Clinical Experiences

Often clinical experiences have been clearly and sometimes narrowly defined for the teacher by the institution. Perhaps the particular patients needed are only available at one place at certain times. It may also be that, because of economic, political, and administrative considerations, alternative clinical experiences are not possible.

However, frequently alternative or optional clinical experiences are available. These can be found by conducting a clinical survey. A clinical survey usually deals with two kinds of data (21): data about the prevailing population factors, socioeconomic problems, and patterns of health within the community; and data about existing health education and welfare agencies, the kinds of facilities that could be utilized, and the availability of specialized consultants.

An initial survey of this type, while time consuming, generates a full assessment of potential clinical experiences. Since the average length of in-patient stay is decreasing, as are in-patient populations, ambulatory services may need to be better utilized as clinical experiences for students. Community clinical experiences or alternative or optional clinical in-hospital experiences give students the opportunity to participate in health-care delivery in a wide range of settings. The clinical survey, which may be as extensive or as brief as the teacher desires, should examine all clinical facilities in the area, as well as all community facilities. Possibly, several teachers might elect to collaborate on gathering survey data.

When planning clinical experiences, it is also important for the teacher to assess the students and the participating faculty. Students' familiarity with the various affiliated institutions can be an influential factor in determining the amount and the type of background preparation and orientation they may need. The teacher also needs to take into account the students' present time schedules in organizing their clinical experiences. Rotating nights may interfere with their day class schedule if both are not considered. Finally, the teacher should determine which courses and experiences students already have had. This is especially important in clinical teaching, where students have an opportunity to integrate and apply what they have learned in courses such as sociology, psychology, and the physical and biological sciences.

In planning the clinical objectives, the teacher needs to consider the results of the student assessment to develop both the minimal competence and the developmental objectives for the clinical experience. Most often clinical experiences involve mastery learning of minimal competence objectives. In general, the clinical objectives involve observational skills, interpersonal skills, skills in judgment making, and motor skills. Once these objectives have been articulated, clinical experiences must be selected to allow students to meet these objectives in a variety of ways.

The teacher responsible for planning clinical experiences needs to consult with other participating teachers to determine the classes or lectures the contributing teachers will be conducting, as well as their specific area of expertise. If there are any time constraints on the participating faculty members' schedules, imposed perhaps by their institutions, these need to be considered. For example, a laboratory supervisor may not be available to students on Monday mornings from 8:00 to 10:00 because of a weekly departmental meeting. It is very important from the beginning to include and encourage participation from all faculty involved to prevent course fragmentation. Because it is common for students to receive content from one teacher and perhaps clinical teaching from another, it is very important for teachers to work closely together, so that the objectives of the course continue to provide its focus and its various learning experiences do not become fragmented.

Selecting Clinical Experiences

In selecting clinical experiences, the teacher may find that grouping clinical objectives into the four areas of observation, interpersonal relationships, decision making, and motor skills will be helpful as a general guide. If the emphasis of the course is on observing, then clinical experiences that encourage this skill should be selected. For example, the first experience might afford students the opportunity to observe a common deviation from normal. Subsequent observations in a different patient population with different implications for care might follow. Finally, clinical situations in which several deviations exist for the student could be provided.

Clinical experiences where students interact not only with patients but also with their families can help in the development of interpersonal skills. Experiences where students also interact with staff can be used for working toward interpersonal objectives as well as for decision-making objectives. Thus, frequently, one clinical experience provides students with a variety of opportunities to work on several objectives.

Since the teacher cannot teach everything, it is important to teach meaningful relationships. In doing this, the continuity and sequencing of activities is very important. Students need to experience repeatedly certain patient behaviors in various situations. Further, they need to begin applying early observations and interventions to eventually more complex and intricate care situations.

The teacher should attempt to provide both long-term and short-term clinical experiences. To achieve an understanding of total patient care, some repetition in experiences is necessary. By not requiring an arbitrary number of clinical experiences, the teacher can require things like three consecutive days of providing care for the same patient or providing care for three postoperative patients.

Once the objectives have been written and the clinical experiences selected, the teacher should begin to plan how the lecture or the content component, if there is one, will be integrated. Specific teaching-learning strategies can be utilized based on the individual needs of the students.

Clinical assignments should *always* be directed at mastery of the objectives, rather than related to the passage of so many clinical days or so many hours. There must also be flexibility in the assignments for students who need more time; likewise, options should be provided for students who need less time. Some teachers inherit courses that have established a certain number of clinical days as a course requirement. Indeed, the decision of number of clinical days may even be an administrative one or one that is established by law. However, these minimum hours are often set much lower than those imposed by teachers within individual courses.

Clinical Schedules

In preparing the clinical schedule, many factors other than the objectives need to be considered. The *availability of instructional help* is one important factor, since students need to have access to the teacher for guidance and assistance. Considering the *clinical area's schedule* is important, because students learn best when they can concentrate on what they are doing. Thus, if students find their care is interrupted frequently by rounds on Monday mornings, perhaps they could be scheduled to be on the units Tuesday mornings instead. A final consideration is the *number of other professionals and other students in the area*. Obviously, the teacher needs to coordinate students' clinical assignments with other disciplines and with the institutions' staffing patterns. Assigning students to teams in which roles are clearly demarcated is one way to maximize learning when a limited number of patients is available (9). While it is often advantageous to have more than one student caring for the patient or to have students from a variety of disciplines care for one client (11), it is never wise to set up a situation in which students must compete for patients. Likewise, students should not be assigned to vastly understaffed areas. It is fine for students to pitch in and help if the unit occasionally needs it, but regular service demands should not be met by students.

In planning the clinical schedule, care should be taken to coordinate classroom activities, clinical activities, and the daily clinical schedule (18). The teacher should not schedule a long clinical day, for example, and then ask students to take a two-hour written examination. Nor should the teacher schedule clinical time for students when grand rounds are held and deny the students an opportunity to participate on rounds.

Whenever possible, pre- and postconferences should be scheduled as part of every clinical day. These can be valuable learning activities. A preclinical conference is an excellent way to help students plan and organize their care. The teacher can be a role model for students and, at the same time, can determine which students will need assistance at approximately what time during that day. This helps the teacher plan how to be available to students as needed. Learning is a post-experience phenomenon (28). Students need to reconstruct their experiences, evaluate their outcomes, and attempt to validate their results. This type of post-learning experience can be carried out by written assignment or, quite effectively, by a short clinical postconference.

Administrative Planning

In planning for clinical learning experiences, the teacher needs to involve administrative staff early in the planning phase. Since student affiliations often require formal contractual agreements, the teacher should begin preparation well in advance. Staff participation in the teaching-learning activities of the students can either be incidental or formal. The exact relationship needs to be clearly spelled out both administratively and by the teacher, so that students are clear about staff participation in student evaluation.

If staff members are going to formally participate in the teaching-learning and evaluation process of the students, they should be actively involved in the course planning and kept informed as the course proceeds. Students should be clearly told the staff members' roles and responsibilities, particularly in relation to course and clinical evaluation. Three-way conferences between staff persons, teachers, and students at designated intervals may be very helpful in charting each student's progress.

Written materials that further describe the clinical learning experiences serve to reinforce the spoken word. These materials can provide structure and security to students who may be anxious and miss some of the information communicated verbally by the teacher. The materials might include the names of staff persons who will be working with the students, as well as the person to report to in case of illness or an emergency. Ideally, information about the clinical learning experience should be a part of the syllabus and should include the clinical objectives, required and suggested readings, and any written assignments, as well as information concerning dress codes and required equipment.

Managing Clinical Experiences

Orientation is an essential part of a clinical learning experience. Students must be shown the physical layout of the institution and must become familiar with its routine procedures. While this is a very necessary activity, it can become boring for the teacher and is perhaps not the best way to spend valuable teacher-student time.

The typical way to handle orientation is for the teacher or a staff person to conduct a tour and then answer questions. While this approach does give the teacher an opportunity to get to know the students, it is often more effective to provide the information in a written, slide-tape, or videotape format. Another method is to take pictures at various points on the tour, mount the pictures, and write explanatory captions next to each. Through use of an independent, media-based approach, the students can, in effect, orient themselves. The hour or so thereby saved can be used to answer questions and begin interacting with students.

Often the use of equipment needs to be demonstrated to students before they begin a specific clinical assignment. One way to conduct demonstrations efficiently is to set up a laboratory containing all the equipment to be used. Students can then try to discover the use of the equipment and, if possible, the means of operating it. In the laboratory, students can practice and reinforce the verbal directions given by the teacher. Certain emergency procedures may need to be mastered, such as cardio-pulmonary-resuscitation or emergency fire evacuation. These too can be demonstrated prior to beginning the experience on specific units.

In managing clinical learning experiences, the teacher has available a multitude of teaching-learning strategies. The selection of these strategies—that is, which strategies should be used with a particular group of students for which objective—depends on the individual situation. The teacher's goal should be to individualize instruction whenever possible.

In general, students need to be helped in planning and organizing care and in applying previously learned principles to the clinical situation. A preconference session may be particularly helpful in accomplishing the former. In addition, written assignments in which students articulate their care and teaching goals are useful both in planning care and in applying concepts and principles to the clinical situation. The goals thus established can serve as a measure for evaluating progress in a postconference; students can discuss why they did what they did and identify the relationship between what they did and what happened. Postconference is also a good time for students to get ongoing feedback about their clinical performance. Clinical pre- and postconferences should be kept small to allow students to consult actively with their peers and their teachers and to receive the help they need.

Objectives related to observational skills should ideally be achieved by moving from simple to complex observations—beginning with patient assignments in which perhaps only one body system is involved and moving eventually to a critically ill patient where observation and monitoring of several body systems is paramount. Observations need to be validated. This can be done by the teacher or a peer making the same observation or, in a laboratory practice situation, by students observing a situation together and then sharing their perceptions of it.

Developing skills of observation in the area of interpersonal interactions can be enhanced by the use of videotapes or audiotapes to record student interactions with patients. The tapes can be reviewed by the student alone or with the teacher, or they can be reviewed in a group with peers. Videotape is a better tool than audiotape, because the nonverbal behaviors that occur can be identified; such identification reinforces students' observational skills. Writing up student-patient interactions, though more time consuming, is another strategy that can be used to help students meet objectives involving interpersonal skills. In addition, weekly clinical supervisory meetings conducted in small groups can assist students in examining the complex issues of interacting with others in the health-care institutions.

To facilitate students' development of sound judgment skills, the teacher needs to provide time for evaluating the care provided within a given time frame and for evaluating whether the care was individualized. Strategies such as a weekly team conference in which the students present their plan of care can be helpful. Students can then receive feedback from peers, professionals of the same or other disciplines, and the teacher.

In assisting students to develop psychomotor skills, the teacher should make extensive use of the practice laboratory (24). Many of the skills can be learned independently through use of excellent media resourses already developed. However, faculty need to be available to answer questions and to evaluate student skill performance levels. It may be possible to have students videotape each other and then critique these tapes before submitting them to the teacher. However, the clinical teacher needs to assume ultimate responsibility for the level of performance of skills acquired in laboratory situations.

Learning psychomotor skills in the laboratory is not sufficient. In order not to forget these skills, students need to engage fairly immediately in a clinical experience (19). Thus, they should be given ample opportunity to repeat these skills in a clinical setting until they are able to perform in the clinic situation as capably as in the laboratory. Students also need the opportunity to apply psychomotor skills in a number of similar situations, followed by a number of dissimilar situations that force them to cope with such things as new equipment or supplies, a new patient condition, or significant changes in the environment. Another potentially effective clinical experience would be for students to teach a psychomotor skill to a patient. Here, the patient would have learning needs similar to those of the student and the opportunity to teach a skill would reinforce the student's mastery of it.

Clinical Evaluation

A variety of written tools can be used in the clinical area. Care plans, process recording, case presentations, case analysis, and case incidence are only a few. Teachers usually have a tool to assess the behaviors specified in the objectives and have some identified times during the course when students receive feedback. Videotape and audiotape are also very useful in helping students evaluate their progress.

Teachers need to know how to observe students directly without interfering in the care they are providing. Since teachers have a responsibility to the patients involved in the clinical program, it may be necessary on occasion to accompany the student to the patient's bedside until the teacher is sure the student can provide the quality of care that is expected.

In the event a teacher feels a student has performed unsafely at the bedside, a colleague should be asked to meet with both the teacher and the student to discuss the specific incident. Then, with the student's consent, the colleague should observe the student clinically to be sure the unsafe behavior is not a misperception—i.e., perhaps the result of a personality conflict between the student and the teacher. However, if the behavior is observed again, the student should be removed from the clinical area.

Based on the two teachers' observations, the next step is to involve the student in a problem-solving session where a plan for remedial learning experiences, usually in the laboratory, is developed. The student should then follow this plan until ready to provide care on the clinical unit again. The teacher should be actively involved with and readily available to the student in the practice laboratory, so the dangerous behavior can be removed. Only when the teacher feels the student has satisfactorily completed the remedial plan should the student resume clinical duties. If the behavior is in the area of judgment making or interpersonal skills, the remedial plan can be more difficult to develop and may require the additional help of a counselor or a learning specialist. Nevertheless, a student who requires this type of tutoring should not come to the clinical unit until the remedial work has corrected the dangerous behaviors. Teachers who attempt to correct these behaviors on the unit usually feel frustrated and find they do not have time to assist and accurately evaluate the other students.

LABORATORY TEACHING

Laboratory experiences provide students with opportunities to engage in various aspects of research, including the use of equipment, the understanding of principles, and participation in the design, analysis, and interpretation of experiments. Since students are exposed to some kind of scientific investigation as a part of most laboratory learning experiences, they can use this experience to further examine and explore their attitudes toward scientific investigation (16).

Two approaches to managing laboratory experiences are available to teachers. The approach they select will depend on their purposes, resources, and students. *Structured laboratory experiences* provide students with carefully formulated instructions and procedures directed at learning the efficient use of equipment or the execution of specific processes. This has been the traditional approach to laboratory management in the health sciences. *Unstructured laboratory experiences* provide students the opportunity to participate in the design and execution of experiments. Students function as members of a research team and are largely responsible for the way an experiment is designed and carried out, as well as for the results their efforts produce. This approach is less common in the health sciences, as it requires the commitment of the teacher's time and laboratory resources to a small number of students.

Structured laboratory experiences, those organized for large groups of students working toward objectives related to operating equipment or instruments or to performing specific procedures, require explicit objectives that are understood by all teachers and students participating in the laboratory. Frequently, when several teachers participate as laboratory advisors, each has a different conception of the correct methods to be followed in the procedure or experiment being conducted. The communication of varying points of view, particularly when precision of execution is required, not only confuses students but may result in their not fully achieving laboratory objectives. Thus, the effectiveness of the laboratory as a learning experience is seriously diminished.

The teacher conducting structured laboratory experiences must be certain the available physical facilities are adequate and that appropriate equipment is available. While students' progress through a procedure or experiment can be impeded by their own mistakes or misunderstandings, it should not be limited by incidental or avoidable obstacles that arise as a result of inadequate or faulty equipment. Students can generally make satisfactory progress, within established time parameters, if encouraged to work at their own speed. They benefit most from the entire experience if left to work on their own, with assistance from the teacher only when needed. Teachers should avoid doing work students can do for themselves (15).

Unstructured laboratory experiences engage students in experiments as members of a research team. Conducted with a small number of students, the unstructured laboratory permits students to participate in the design and execution of experiments, thereby immersing them in the theory and practice of scientific investigation. This approach promotes discovery learning and, while it requires more of a commitment of the teacher's time and resources, it should be considered for inclusion as part of any total laboratory sequence.

A basic framework for students' self-directed work in an unstructured laboratory experience, found to be effective as a teaching-learning strategy (25), follows the scientific approach to problem solving through experimentation. Teachers and students first discuss together the objectives of a research project; each student or small group of students then selects one problem to pursue as a means of achieving the overall objectives of the project. After conducting a search through the primary and secondary literature sources, students establish working hypotheses and plan the strategy they will follow in conducting their experiment. They then consult with the teacher as needed in establishing appropriate methodology and data collection procedures, and work independently in executing their experiment or project. The teacher is available during this time for assistance, but avoids interfering with student progress. Students are responsible for observations, note keeping, and the analysis of data. Because the process of scientific investigation is the focal point of the unstructured laboratory, and because discovery learning is encouraged in students, students must be prepared to conclude their research with objectivity—i.e., they must be prepared to accept expected results as well as the lack of expected results.

The unstructured laboratory experience is perhaps most appropriate for advanced courses and advanced students. It can also be appropriate, however, for large groups of beginning students, if the large group can be broken into smaller units and if resources and the assistance of other teachers or laboratory assistants are available.

A variation of the unstructured laboratory, which includes some elements of the structured experience, can also be used with large groups of students. This approach is based on the concept of modules. A sequence of laboratory experiences is divided into a logical grouping of subjects, each of which is further divided into a set of specific learning objectives (1). This procedure is similar to that used for developing learning packages; laboratory experiences are arranged so that students may work at them independently. Each student receives a laboratory manual that includes a schedule of learning objectives, appropriate notebooks or other recording mechanisms and materials, and administrative directions. Students then conduct specific laboratory experiences, either in small groups or independently, following preestablished learning experiences directed at the achievement of specific objectives.

Effective laboratory teaching requires the explication of learning objectives and the clear demonstration of the relationship between the objectives, the experience itself, and the other course activities of the students. Students who understand the importance and the relevance of the laboratory experience are likely to involve themselves actively in its execution.

In managing learning in the structured and unstructured laboratory, it may be possible to vary both the approaches to assignments and the amount of time that students have to complete them. There may be budgetary constraints that do not allow the laboratory to be open for extra hours to students, in which case the teacher needs to be most efficient in the use of available time. Students might be able, for example, to check out simple equipment, which they can then use outside the laboratory to master specific skills, so that valuable laboratory time is freed for other activities. Students might also be given information and guidelines for beginning the design of experiments at home, so that they are ready to implement their designs as soon as they enter the laboratory.

In managing the laboratory experience, the teacher also needs to know when to structure an experience for a student, when to intervene if the student is making a mistake, and when to allow a student the time for discovery that can lead to learning. This is a highly specialized skill and teachers should not assume that it comes easily or automatically with time. Certainly experience contributes to the teacher's expertise and the ability to manage a wide variety of learning-related behaviors; however, the laboratory teacher needs to try new strategies in the laboratory continually, attempting always to improve its quality as a learning experience for students.

REFERENCES

1. BICKLEY, HARMON C., ROBERT P. RAPP, AND CHARLES A. WALTON. "A Course in Pathology for Pharmacy Students. I. Rationale and Description." *American Journal of Pharmaceutical Education* 37 (1973): 620–626.

2. COLLINS, BARRY E. *Social Psychology: Social Influence, Attitude Change, Group Processes, and Prejudice.* Reading, Mass.: Addison-Wesley, 1970.

3. DAVIS, JAMES H. *Group Performance.* Reading, Mass.: Addison-Wesley, 1970.

4. GAGE, NATHANIEL L., AND DAVID C. BERLINER. *Educational Psychology.* Chicago: Rand McNally, 1975.

5. GALLAGHER, JAMES B., JR. "An Evaluation of the Transfer of Information by Printed Materials without a Formal Lecture." *Journal of Dental Education* 34 (1970): 59–66.

6. GULLEY, HOLBERT E. *Discussion, Conference, and Group Process.* 2d ed. New York: Holt, Rinehart and Winston, 1968.

7. HARE, A. PAUL. *Handbook of Small Group Research.* 2d ed. New York: Free Press, 1976.

8. HYMAN, RONALD T. *Ways of Teaching.* Philadelphia: Lippincott, 1970.

9. HYMOVICH, DEBRA. "Coordinated Student Learning." *Nursing Outlook* 18 (1970): 62–64.

10. JUSTIN, JOSEPH, AND WALTER H. MAIS. *College Teaching: Its Practice and Potential.* New York: Harper and Brothers, 1956.

11. MASON, ELIZABETH, AND JOHN PARASCANDOLA. "Preparing Tomorrow's Health Care Team." *Nursing Outlook* 20 (1972): 728–731.

12. McCREA, MARION W., AND ERNEST A. SWANSON, JR. "Are Formal Lectures Really Necessary?" *Journal of Dental Education* 33 (1969): 424–431.

13. McLEISH, JOHN. *The Lecture Method.* Cambridge, England: Cambridge Institute of Education, 1968.

14. McLEISH, JOHN, WAYNE MATHESON, AND JAMES PARK.. *The Psychology of the Learning Group.* London, England: Hutchinson University Library, 1973.

15. MILLER, GEORGE E. et al. *Teaching and Learning in Medical School.* Cambridge, Mass.: Harvard University Press, 1962.

16. NEDELSKY, LEO. *Science Teaching and Testing.* New York: Harcourt, Brace and World, 1965.

17. O'SHEA, HELEN. "Reinforcing Clinical Study." *Nursing Outlook* 18 (1970): 59–61.

18. PEARSON, BETTY D. "Considerations for Student Clinical Assignments." *Journal of Nursing Education* 16 (1977): 3–5.

19. PORTER, ROBERT M. "Relationship of Participation to Satisfaction in Small Group Discussions." *Journal of Educational Research* 59 (1965): 128–132.

20. POTTER, DAVID, AND MARTIN P. ANDERSON. *Discussion: A Guide to Effective Practice.* Belmont, Ca.: Wadsworth, 1963.

21. SCHWEER, JEAN, E., AND KRISTINE M. GEBBIE. *Creative Teaching in Clinical Nursing.* 3d ed. St. Louis: C. V. Mosby, 1976.

22. SOMMER, ROBERT. "Classroom Ecology." *Journal of Applied Behavioral Science* 3 (1967): 489–503.

23. STUCK, DEAN L., AND RICHARD P. MANATT. "A Comparison of Audiotutorial and Lecture Methods of Teaching." *Journal of Educational Research* 63 (1970): 414–418.

24. SULLIVAN, KAREN et al. "From Learning Modules to Clinical Practice." *Nursing Outlook* 25 (1977): 319–321.

25. SZINAI, S. S., AND N. SZINAI. "A Meaningful Experience in Laboratory Investigation." *American Journal of Pharmaceutical Education* 40 (1976): 248–250.

26. THOMPSON, RALPH. "Legitimate Lecturing." *Improving College and University Teaching* 22 (1974): 163–164.

27. WARE, JOHN E., AND REED G. WILLIAMS. "The Doctor Fox Effect: A Study of Lecturer Effectiveness and Ratings of Instruction." *Journal of Medical Education* 50 (1975): 149–156.

28. WIEDENBACH, ERNESTINE. *Meeting the Realities in Clinical Teaching.* New York: Springer, 1971.

𝒪

PERSONALIZED INSTRUCTION

Individualized instruction is an educational catchword used to describe a variety of strategies and methods used at various levels of education. Its strict definition implies that one-to-one instruction takes place between a teacher and student, so that the individual needs and interests of each student are recognized and accommodated. If teachers were to pursue the requirements of individualized instruction rigidly, they would diagnose each student's learning needs and interests and then develop and implement specific instructional approaches for each student based on the results of these diagnoses. Each student's progress would require careful monitoring; the teacher would have to be flexible enough to schedule remedial or advanced work for each student when needed.

In practice, individualized instruction is infrequently implemented. Time constraints, large numbers of students scheduled into classes, and the lack of sufficient administrative and resource support make it an unfeasible approach. A more appropriate and realistic approach is personalized instruction. Personalized instruction can be conducted on a one-to-many basis as well as on a one-to-one basis. It entails identifying student needs and interests and helping students to do the same, as well as providing one or more alternative teaching-learning strategies from which students can choose to achieve specific learning objectives.

Strategies for the management of personalized instruction can be viewed along a continuum. At one end are learning packages, a strategy that can be used with a large number of students to provide some degree of personalization. In the middle of the continuum is contingency contracting, an approach usually used with smaller numbers of students which provides an even greater degree of personalization. Tutoring, usually for remedial purposes, is at the other end of the continuum. It is highly personalized and can be conducted on a one-to-one basis or with very small groups of students. The degree of teacher involvement with students and the degree of personalization of instruction increases across the continuum from learning packages to tutoring.

Differences in these strategies for personalizing instruction do not imply that they are mutually exclusive. It is possible, for example, to tutor a student who is also utilizing learning packages in the course or unit. The teacher needs to be aware of the potential of these various strategies and be able to choose among them according to personal time commitments and student needs.

LEARNING PACKAGES

Learning packages can be used with a large number of students to personalize learning. It may be possible to develop a learning package for a lecture, so that the student has at least two options: either to listen to a tape of the lecture or to attend the lecture. Or, the learning package for a lecture may be more extensive and more personal. It may contain a tape of the lecture, several reading assignments, a simulation game, and programmed instruction that can be used by the students to achieve specific objectives. In this way, several learning styles and needs can be accommodated in a large course at the same time.

Another possibility is to eliminate some lectures and replace them with learning packages, thereby allowing the teacher more time and energy to personalize instruction for students. The time freed from lecture preparation can then be used to deal with students having difficulty progressing in the course. It can also provide the teacher with time to plan for including more learning options. For example, the teacher may design some type of group interaction for class time or may even cluster students within groups to further personalize instruction. Any strategy that allows the teacher to increase the time available to transact with students—i.e., answer individual questions, as well as problem solve with them—is also increasing the personalization of instruction.

Most teachers would like to be able to offer their students a variety of ways of achieving course objectives, but do not have the necessary time to plan these options. Developing course material and finding new clinical facilities that can be used as alternate learning sources require a great deal of the teacher's time. Learning packages can be used to help the teacher manage a course more efficiently and effectively and can thus provide more time for the teacher to attempt to personalize instruction within the course.

Students should be oriented to the purpose and use of learning packages at the beginning of a course or unit. They should be made aware that the choice of approach they make will be both viable and valuable to their progress toward specific objectives.

Orientation begins in the initiation phase of the group life of the course. Rather than beginning a course with learning packages—a strategy that some students may not have encountered previously—teachers should schedule them for the working phase of the course. As part of the process of establishing trust between teacher and students, the teacher should explain to the students during this time that learning packages have been designed for their use; that lecture attendance is not necessary to "get all the information" needed for a test; and that they will not miss important information by choosing an alternative strategy. This explanation will be borne out by the first self-assessment accompanying a learning package, for it will reflect objectives that could have been achieved through attending a lecture, completing a programmed instruction sequence, or listening to an audiotape. With this orientation and preparation, students proceed into the working phase knowing that the alternative strategies available to them are "for real" and are there to be used as they see fit.

CONTINGENCY CONTRACTING

Contingency contracting employs systematic motivation techniques in a personalized instructional setting. By using contingency contracting, it is possible for the teacher systematically to reward desired behavior in a student each time it occurs. It is also possible to negotiate with a student in advance regarding the framework within which learning is to take place. Both of these approaches can encourage motivation in students.

On the continuum of personalized instruction, contingency contracting is the strategy most appropriate for a small group of learners who do not need remedial tutoring but who may have difficulty progressing within a course. This difficulty may stem from such factors as inability to self-pace, absences due to illness, or motivational or attitudinal problems.

It may appear that developing contracts with students who have difficulty pacing their learning represents the teacher doing the pacing for the student. However, the objective of contingency contracts is to shift students to self-management, so that eventually they assume responsibility for their own motivation and learning.

While the teacher helps the student develop the contract, it is the student who actually manages it. Thus contingency contracting is making an agreement with a student in which the outcome is agreed to be dependent on the student's performance (2).

Teachers often use contracts with students on an informal basis. To say to a student, "If you do X and Y, I'll do Z and you will pass the course," is essentially a contract. However, because this agreement is not structured and formally written, there can be subsequent misinterpretations on the part of both student and teacher. The contingency contract, a written agreement between the teacher and the student that follows certain guidelines, avoids this difficulty.

Five guidelines should be followed when using contingency contracts with students (2). The first is that the *reward should be immediate.* This is particularly important when the student is just beginning to learn about contracting. Thus, if the contract's ultimate objective is to have the student pass a semester course successfully, it is better to have four four-week contracts than one sixteen-week contract, so that rewards are more immediate.

The second guideline is to *reward frequently with small amounts rather than once with one large amount.* Within a four-week contract, outcomes and rewards should be identified for each week. The rewards should be contingent on demonstration of adequate performance of the behavior and not, for example, on the passage of time. Thus, instead of saying, "Will be able to perform routine urinalysis," the desired behavior is broken down into, "Will be able to measure the specific gravity of urine."

Initial contracts should call for and reward small approximations of the targeted behavior. The focus should be on describing small, simple-to-perform approximations of the final desired behavior, rather than on large units that may be more difficult, or even impossible, for the student to perform satisfactorily.

The contract should call for and reward accomplishment rather than obedience. The objective of contracts is to help students develop self-management skills of learning and develop the motivation to learn. It is very important that the student not view the contract as a decree from the teacher—i.e., "You do what I say and you'll receive this reward." This approach favors dependence and obedience. The contract should be an agreement on behavior outcomes; when these behaviors are achieved, the rewards automatically follow.

The final guideline is *reward the performance after it occurs.* While this seems obvious, the reverse sometimes occurs. For example, if the student's goal is to become a nurse and one evidence of this is bathing a patient, then the reward for learning how to bathe a patient is the actual opportunity to perform the procedure.

Five characteristics apply to the process of contracting (2). The contract must be fair, clear, honest, and positive, and contracting as a method must be used systematically.

It is assumed the contract will be fair, clear, and honest. But the teacher may be tempted to use terms like "I will not do X, if you will do Y." This is a negative contract and involves the threat of punishment. Such contracts are unproductive, since they do not encourage independence.

When using contracting, care should be taken not to reward undesirable behaviors. The best way to eliminate unwanted behaviors is to make certain that they are *never* reinforced. If a student habitually turns in assignments late, this behavior should never be rewarded, even when it becomes significantly diminished.

Teachers sometimes feel that rewarding students is unethical; they believe adults should not need rewards to learn. However, the fact remains that adult learners who are having difficulty learn better and are more willing to continue learning if rewards follow difficult activities. While contracting can be done with groups, its most frequent use is with particular students who are having trouble progressing in the course and who need some kind of personalized instruction.

The objective is to help students develop their own motivation and self-management of learning.

A contract must be stated in simple language. It must specify exactly the amount of work required of a student, as well as the reward to be received. In addition, the "beginning" and "end" of the contract should be clearly established. Although an end may be difficult to describe for a health science professional, since learning is seen as a dynamic, lifelong process, a clearly defined end point can be a significant factor in increasing the motivation of a student who is experiencing difficulty in progressing.

The next step for the teacher is to define exactly what constitutes a reward for a given student. In general, there are two types of rewards—one of them purely entertaining and the other a preferred academic activity. What may be a reward for one student may not be considered desirable by another. One student may want to pass the course so that a summer session can be used for a vacation, while another may want to pass the course in order to continue in the normal school rotation. A reward might be a day off to go shopping or the opportunity to do advanced work within the course.

In attempting to select a reinforcement or reward, it is helpful to ask: What would the student rather be doing? What rewards are actively being sought? The student is the best source of information on what is personally reinforcing at any one time.

Progress checks are very important and a valuable component of the contingency contract. They provide the teacher with a clear indication of the student's completion of the task assignment and they also indicate to the student how much progress has been made. This progress check can be a short weekly or daily meeting.

It may be necessary to either lengthen or shorten the contract. Contracts can malfunction for a variety of reasons. Certain external factors outside of the student's control may make it impossible for the student to fulfill the contract in the time allotted. In this case, the contract can be lengthened. Or, if the student has found that the contract can be met more quickly, the contract can be shortened. Each situation must be judged individually and the teacher must determine if the contract should be renegotiated. Having the option to renegotiate provides the teacher with flexibility and a further opportunity to personalize instruction for the student.

TUTORING

A student's learning difficulties or academic failures can generally be attributed to some attitudinal or motivational factor or to some deficiency in the student's learning background or preparation for a course. Whatever the reason, students with difficulties can be assisted through tutoring.

Tutoring is a form of personalized instruction that works well with students who have motivational or attitudinal problems, because it provides a structured approach to learning and a schedule of feedback and rewards. Tutoring can also be used with students who have some deficiency in their educational background. Such instruction generally takes place on a one-to-one basis.

Difficulty in learning can usually be traced to a student's lack of some prerequisite (1). The prerequisite can be content related, such as an inability to grasp facts or principles that are basic to more advanced content, or it can be skill related, such as an inability to read or study efficiently.

The exact nature of a student's deficiency must be diagnosed before tutoring can take place. The diagnosis begins with the observation that a particular student is missing content prerequisites, is having difficulty meeting objectives, or cannot keep up with the rest of the class. Observation can be accomplished informally by the teacher or formally through some form of pretesting or diagnostic testing. Results of the observation indicate what type of tutoring would be most effective. Diagnostic activities continue as tutoring progresses; their purpose is to indicate to the teacher exactly how the student is or is not progressing.

Both teachers and nonteachers can tutor students. Nonteachers may be educational specialists or faculty or graduate assistants. They can be most helpful in working with students who have study-skill or reading problems. Given the appropriate preparation, they can also tutor students with deficiencies in educational backgrounds.

The first requirement of a tutor is affective in nature. Tutors must be able to create a relaxed environment for learning, yet at the same time indicate to the student the need for accomplishing specific objectives. Students in need of tutoring generally have no problem recognizing their deficiency; however, because their learning difficulty tends to set them apart from their peers, they appreciate a relaxed learning environment and a nonthreatening relationship with someone who intends to help them.

General procedures to be followed in developing a tutoring schedule for students are similar to those associated with programmed instruction. A content program, specific to what is to be taught, is first established. The content program is divided into a series of parts of steps through which the student will proceed with the tutor. Provisions for feedback based on student responses given during the program are included. A student can then progress to another lesson, repeat a lesson, or omit a lesson, depending on whether or not mastery has been demonstrated (3).

The content of the tutoring program is similar to that presented in a classroom situation, e.g., a lecture. Its presentation is different, however, because the tutor's purpose is to make certain that the student knows the content covered. The presentation of the program is characterized by a loop process which begins when the student is presented with a problem. If the student responds incorrectly, the error is noted and the problem, question, or statement is repeated by the tutor along with the correct answer.

Students involved in this type of tutoring system are generally required to meet a 90 percent mastery level, i.e., they should provide 90 percent or better correct responses to the given problems, questions, or statements. If they meet this level, they go on to more advanced programs; if they do not meet it, they are required to repeat the lesson or its equivalent.

The tutoring process can be effective for bringing students with learning difficulties to a desired level of performance. It has been shown to be more effective and more efficient in this regard than traditional teaching methods (3). Because of its potential effectiveness, and because it can be conducted by teachers and nonteachers, tutoring as a strategy for personalizing instruction should be given serious consideration by teachers seeking a means to assist students with learning difficulties.

REFERENCES

1. GAGNE, ROBERT M. *The Conditions of Learning.* New York: Holt, Rinehart, and Winston, 1965.

2. HOMME, LLOYD. *How to Use Contingency Contracting in the Classroom.* Champaign, Ill.: Research Press, 1969.

3. ROSENBAUM, PETER S. *Peer-Mediated Instruction.* New York: Teachers College Press, 1973.

10
GROUP SKILLS

Group teaching involves students communicating among themselves as well as with the teacher. The crucial difference between group teaching and traditional teaching is that the process occurs between and among the students and the teacher, regardless of the particular strategy being used. For example, simulation games involve the use of groups and the group process as well as seminars.

Some teachers believe that the "best" learning occurs in a one-to-one relationship where the student has free and exclusive access to the teacher. Certainly in some learning situations, such as tutorials, preceptorships, or postgraduate study, this is true. However, this type of learning situation is not the most common. Usually students in the health sciences are taught in large lecture courses and small clinical groups.

Due to increasing enrollments, low student-teacher ratios are no longer economically feasible. Thus many teachers are experiencing pressure to accommodate more students in their courses without sacrificing their standards. This situation can provide a positive impetus for teachers to investigate alternative strategies, such as games and learning packages. These strategies are successful, however, only if the teacher has the necessary skills to implement them.

Group skills are necessary not only for traditional strategies, but also for many of the strategies described in Unit 2—specifically, media, simulation games, and learning packages. These strategies either require group skills themselves (e.g., simulations) or require small-group experiences as adjunct activities (e.g., learning packages).

The teacher who is familiar with group theory and has consciously developed group skills is able to *consistently* plan and lead group learning experiences and *competently* handle common group problems. By developing this set of teaching skills, the teacher is able to remove the chance factor from the teaching situation and maximize opportunities for learning.

There are advantages and disadvantages to small- or large-group experiences. First, by being taught in groups and seeing several teachers using different leadership styles, health science students begin to learn how to lead groups themselves. Learning experiences where students have a chance to study groups, lead groups themselves, and receive feedback on their skills are more common now in health science curricula. Either a specific group course may be offered or required or group content may be integrated in an existing course, such as a course in ward management. With increasing costs in health care, it is becoming more important for future practitioners to be able to conduct health care activities in groups. For example, it is more economical to teach diabetics how to regulate their diets in groups than it would be to teach each person individually.

A commonly shared belief among health care professionals is that certain health-care activities occur "best" or "most effectively" in a one-to-one relationship, specifically personal counseling and clinical supervision. This notion can be challenged, since often the criteria used to determine if it is "good" or "effective" is the health care practitioner's comfort or the client's comfort. This comfort is often related to whether the learning situation is a new or unfamiliar one. Certain learning can occur effectively in both situations. Research needs to be conducted to provide the health care professional with information about when groups are most effective for what types of clients. Currently research in this area is lacking. Often economics or the clinical situation dictates whether the health care practitioner uses an individual or a group approach.

The myth of the effectiveness of the one-to-one relationship also exists for the health science teacher and the student, particularly for such activities as clinical evaluations and supervision. Again, this is often related to the comfort of the teacher and the student; discussing personal assets and limitations in front of peers in a small-group setting can be uncomfortable.

However, using this one-to-one approach has some disadvantages. The student may not be able to "hear" what the teacher is saying because of an interpersonal conflict or because the teacher is viewed as an authority figure. In managing this type of situation, peers can be very helpful in validating feedback the teacher is giving or in challenging this feedback when it is incorrect. Evaluating students in groups can also demonstrate to them that the difficulty they are experiencing is "normal." This is often not possible when the feedback occurs behind closed doors in a one-to-one evaluation session. But when it occurs in front of a group of peers who are obviously struggling with the same problem areas, it can be quite helpful.

In general, then, group activities encourage students to share, to problem solve, and to begin learning how to consult with one another. This particular skill is important to the continued growth of the student as a graduate practitioner.

Group experiences are particularly important for developmental objectives, since the teacher is able to transact with the student directly. Students can also be clustered in several groups according to the specific objectives they are learning. This arrangement can be particularly useful, since many of these objectives involve developing the communication or interactional skills of the student, skills vital to the health care professional.

ASSESSING GROUP SKILLS

Some teachers have had formal instruction in group theory, but need help in applying the theory to teaching in groups. Other teachers may have had a great deal of practical experience, but lack the theoretical framework to interpret, predict, and plan for group learning experiences. In assessing the teacher's level of skill development in working with groups, it is helpful if a colleague or peer with group expertise can observe the teacher in action.

The assessment should be threefold. The peer reviewer should: (1) interpret the group process for the teacher in terms of the specific session and in terms of the life of the group; (2) evaluate whether and how the goals were reached; and (3) describe the assets and limitations of the leader. In a postsession the peer reviewer and the teacher should compare their observations and interpretations.

It is most helpful if the peer reviewer and the teacher can agree in advance on a framework to use in interpreting the process of the group and in evaluating the teacher's effectiveness in accomplishing the objectives of the group. The following framework is one of many that can be used to assess the teacher's current skills.

In assessing a group, it is helpful to think of the life of the group as consisting of three phases. These phases are summarized in Table 10.1. They are the initiation phase, working phase, and termination phase. In the *initiation phase*, students are oriented to a course or unit and begin to develop trust. In the *working phase,* the group engages in problem solving. Finally, in the *termination phase,* the students withdraw and separate from one another.

Initiation Phase

In this phase, the teacher defines the objectives for the group session and facilitates discussion intended to help members develop trust in one another by testing out certain behaviors in the group. Thus, the role of the teacher is to *orient* the student to what is expected of them and how they should accomplish this; and to *facilitate trust* in the group, both among the students and between the students and the teacher.

It is essential in a teaching-learning situation for the teacher to orient the students clearly to the objectives of the group. For example, during a lecture or a laboratory experience, students may be meeting to increase their applied diagnostic skills by critiquing a case study presented to them by one of the group mem-

Table 10.1.
Summary of Group Phases

Group Phases	Goals	Group Strategies	Leader Behaviors
Initiation	Orient group. Facilitate trust.	Introduces self and students. Describes objectives and purpose of group. Orients group to time limitations and behavior expected of each student. Encourages questions and discussion of group activities.	Reduces group anxiety. Sets limits. Deals with anger without becoming defensive. Displays trust.
Working	Encourage problem solving.	Presents group with problem-solving situations, games, or opportunities. Intervenes only to facilitate problem solving.	Shares control with group. Directs problem solving.
Termination	Initiate termination. Facilitate separation.	Initiates discussion of termination. Allows for group regression and encourages reminiscing and expressions of warmth, anger, and depression. Accepts and encourages distancing devices and final separation.	Facilitates and accepts angry feelings. Accepts warm feelings. Accepts regression. Accepts separation.

bers; or to examine by way of a group simulation exercise the implications of long-term residential treatment for alcoholics and its effects on the family structure. Too often the objectives for the group have not been clearly defined and the teacher has only a vague idea of what is to be accomplished and how. Since this information is not clear to the students, valuable learning time can be lost and unnecessary anxiety can be generated in the group.

Orientation to the purposes of the group, based on the teacher's ability to establish and communicate the goals of the session, is very important in the initiation phase. The objective of the group may be to give students a chance to ask the teacher questions or to apply the information they have learned outside of class in real clinical situations. Whatever the objective, the teacher should be sure to stay on course and not stray from the group's stated purpose. If, for example, the teacher implies that the objective is to answer questions, time should not be used to assess students' ability to problem solve.

The orientation should also alert the students, as much as possible, to the strategies planned for accomplishing the objectives. Certainly there needs to be room for spontaneity and the teacher can clearly revise strategies as appropriate.

However, if the objectives for the group are to be met through lecture-discussion, or by a case-study method, or by using a simulation game, the students should be informed in advance so they can be prepared for the session.

Testing, or challenging, is a way that students discover for themselves whether they can *trust* the teacher and each other. Students challenge each other's statements to see if opinions and behaviors remain constant. Students who seem to mean what they say prompt trust, while students who change opinions or behavior often usually generate anxiety and mistrust in the group until group members feel they know them and can account for these changes.

Trust and intimacy among students always precedes any attempt to know and trust the teacher. Once each group member has tested the other group members, then the group will, as a whole, admit the teacher into the group. This often occurs at the end of the initiation phase and just before the working phase. Testing of the teacher may take the form of students challenging a rule (to see if the teacher really means what is said), turning in a paper late, or coming to class late. This behavior is often unconscious and automatic. Once students have developed this very important sense of trust, they can go into the working phase and work more productively on the course objectives.

Teachers also "test" students. Initially, a teacher may try to develop a sense of intimacy with the group and become personally acquainted with the particular individuals within the group. Usually just before the working phase begins, the teacher seems to find it difficult or impossible to get to class on time. This is a form of unconscious testing in that the teacher is very responsive to how the students react to the teachers' being late. Do they leave or begin without the teacher? Or do they stay, but ignore the teacher's arrival?

Thus the role of the teacher in the initiation phase is to orient the students and to facilitate trust within the group. The more quickly this can be done, the better, for it serves to minimize the friction and anxiety in the group. When students test, it is often easy to respond to the testing behavior with defensive behavior. However, the ability to interpret this behavior as being necessary for the group of a particular student is essential, since the goal is to establish trust quickly and move on to the next stage, the working phase.

Working Phase

The role of the teacher in the working phase is to facilitate student problem solving to help them accomplish the objectives of the course. To do this, the teacher carefully plans strategies that are in harmony with the life of the group and the objective of the group. This is the most fruitful phase of the group and the teacher is much less active now. A skilled teacher is able to facilitate problem solving with a minimum of direct involvement. It is a time when the students can actively try out and experience themselves in the group.

In the working phase, both teacher and students usually feel good about the group's activity. Their specific activities at this time are difficult to describe, because while most groups tend to initiate and terminate in similar ways, the working-phase activities can be vastly different. They are dependent on a particular purpose of the group.

During this phase, the teacher can work on developmental goals for each student—for example, help a shy student work on interviewing skills. Thus, at this time, the teacher is likely to consider the needs of individual students in planning group strategies.

Toward the end of the working phase, the teacher should begin to prepare the students for termination of the group.

Termination Phase

The role of the teacher in the termination phase is to help students prepare for the end of the course or unit by reviewing their progress and growth. During this phase, both negative and positive feelings about the course are expressed and students begin to distance themselves from one another in preparation for termination. The teacher needs to be able to deal with students' denial, anger, and depression and eventually lead them to a comfortable separation from other students, the teacher, and the course.

The process of termination is frequently neglected by teachers. Many argue that students don't really have enough time to get involved in a course or feel close to other class members; thus, these teachers do not see the need to deal with end-of-course feelings. Students become involved in different degrees, but to say they do not react to finishing the course is both an understatement and a valuable learning opportunity missed. At this time, teachers can help students begin to learn how to terminate relationships and handle change in their own lives.

Some teachers are uncomfortable with the warm, tender feelings frequently expressed during termination. Many of the behaviors at the end of the course are similar to those at the beginning. Students may need to be reoriented to the final course expectations and they may also engage in testing behaviors again—e.g., being late for class or late with assignments. In the termination phase, these behaviors serve to distance the students from the teacher and the students from each other.

Table 10.1 provides the basis for assessing one's own group leadership skills. Both a colleague and the students in the group should be asked to evaluate the teacher according to the criteria provided here. The results should prove to be a fairly accurate assessment of current skills.

DEVELOPING GROUP SKILLS

Developing group skills can be done in a wide variety of ways. Formal courses are offered in both theory and practice of groups. Usually the course has a specific orientation, such as instructional groups, counseling groups, or psychotherapeutic groups. Many of the principles are the same, but the application of these principles can be very different. For example, teaching French to adults in small groups is different from teaching pediatric nursing in small groups. What often makes the difference is the significance of the behavioral change involved. In the French course, students are expected to develop new communicative and syntactical skills. While students might be very involved, the emotional impact is less than asking a student to be able to provide total patient care for an adolescent with severe burns. To use group process to teach content and to facilitate and synthesize learning for students requires a thorough understanding of and skills in group dynamics, as well as skill in interpreting human behavior.

Often group skills are learned and practiced by the teacher in the process of teaching. Team teaching or peer evaluation of current skills can be very helpful in developing new skills. While this is not as structured an approach to developing new skills as is a formal course, it is often the most practical way.

Courses and practice in interpreting human behavior also can be very helpful. Learning is a growth experience and the more sensitive the teacher can be to the developmental crises of the students, the more likely it is that learning experiences will coincide rather than conflict with the growth of the student.

Increasing one's self-awareness through self-reflection is necessary to becoming an effective teacher. Insight into personal assets and limitations makes it easier to extend a part of the self to a student who is growing, learning, and developing new behaviors. Insight gives the teacher power and control. The threat of a new student discovering the teacher's imperfections disappears when the teacher has already recognized and accepted these flaws. Such recognition makes it possible to be honest with students.

By the same token, it is very difficult to plan and implement interpersonal learning activities such as small groups if the teacher is not aware of the students' personal assets or limitations. For example, to know that silence is anxiety provoking for group members, and to further recognize that the teacher tends to step in to fill the silence, is an important insight. By filling the silence, the teacher deprives the students of becoming involved and causes them to depend on this intervention when there is silence. With this type of insight, the teacher can try new strategies to eliminate the problem by determining why the silence is so anxiety provoking and what the group can do to alleviate this situation.

It is, of course, unwise for the teacher to become so concerned with the interpersonal aspects of group dynamics as to lose sight of learning strategies and course objectives. It is also possible to give too much of the self to students and to become personally depleted. A teacher must both give and take from students and should expect to grow and learn along with the students. The message should be clear that the teacher is willing to get involved with the class, but also expects to learn from the students. By removing many of the issues of control and traditional classroom role behaviors, the teacher can encourage the uniqueness of each student to surface.

Knowing when to use a particular group strategy is a skill most teachers want to further develop. Too often, a variety of group strategies is not utilized; instead traditional strategies are maintained, such as the question-answer, case-presentation, or presentation-discussion methods. While these can be very effective, efficient strategies, they are often limiting in the amount of group process they encourage.

Games, simulations, and various other planned group activities involve much more group process among the students and between the teacher and the group. But the decision of when to use what activity is a very complex one. The activity must enable students to meet course objectives and, at the same time, must facilitate the specific goals of the group, depending on the phase of life of the group. For example, while both a game and a case study might be appropriate strategies for a set of objectives, the game may be more appropriate than the case if the group is in the initiation phase of group life. That is, if the case study requires the group to problem solve as a whole, then it is best to delay this activity until the working phase, when people know each other and can share and problem solve as a group. If such a strategy were used in the initiation phase, testing might occur or one group member might monopolize the conversation. On the other hand, some group case-study strategies are very structured and are quite effective in giving students a chance to know each other better by working together on a common problem.

Thus the choice or choices of group strategies is critical. It must be based on an accurate interpretation of the stage of the group. There are several written resources to help the teacher with strategies (see especially Pfeiffer in the Unit 3 bibliography), but the teacher may also want to observe other teachers using a group approach or participate in a group where a variety of strategies is used.

Each group session should reflect the teacher's preparation. It is as important for a teacher to review the process of the last group session and how the current session's objectives are to be accomplished as it is to review lecture notes before a lecture. The strategies should be prepared and perhaps even piloted on a small group before they are used with the students.

The life of the group, as well as each session, has three phases and the teacher should evaluate group progress each week so that strategies appropriate to each phase can be implemented at the proper time. Thus, by the middle of the course, the group as a whole should trust one another sufficiently to be able to problem solve. If the group cannot, the teacher should assess why and plan and implement group activities designed to nurture group trust. Each session should also allow for a few minutes of initiation phase, longer initially but shorter by the end of the course, in which students are told the objectives for that session.

The teacher must be adept at dealing with two types of behaviors in groups: anxiety and testing behavior. Anxiety—of the group in general or of specific members—can occur at any time, but is most common at the beginning, before students know each other. At this time, students often do not know what to expect or what is expected of them. Initially this anxiety can be dealt with by the teacher providing structured experiences and a general orientation; however, anxiety at a later point in the group indicates some type of conflict and the teacher needs to be able to interpret it and respond to it appropriately. In some instances, the teacher may choose to allow a high level of anxiety to continue if this anxiety is currently facilitating the group process (e.g., problem solving).

The beginning of the course is also an anxiety provoking time for the teacher. It is important that the teacher recognize how this anxiety affects the ability to lead a learning group, so that this anxious behavior can be examined and ultimately resolved.

Testing behaviors are common in groups. They are most frequent in the initiation phase, but they can also occur any time. Many students view the teacher as an authority/parent figure, and thus they may be unconsciously acting out their conflict with authority figures in class. The teacher should avoid becoming defensive and should deal with the conflict in the here and now by helping the student understand the basis for this response to authority. This is an important insight for any student preparing to work in the health care field.

Two other common problems often surface in the group setting. The first is silence in a group; the second is anger. Silence can mean very different things depending on when it occurs in the life of the group and what the current issue is. It may be a hostile, testing silence, in which the students are testing the teacher to see what happens when they do not do what is required. Or, it may merely be an indication that the group is thinking. Alternatively, it could be a depressed silence indicating an inability of the group to talk about and deal with certain difficult feelings; or it could be the group's way of silencing a student who talks all the time. Thus, the teacher must develop skill in interpreting the meaning of silence, so as to know when and how to intervene.

Anger can be a very difficult feeling to confront, since it is very hard for most teachers to be honest about this emotion. Some teachers discourage any expression of real feeling in their groups, implying that such emotions are "inappropriate" for the classroom, while others encourage students to act out their feelings and may find themselves worrying about losing control in the group.

Honesty in groups is paramount. The expressions "I disagree," "I'm afraid," or "I can't tolerate that" should be allowed and respected. Health science students as adult learners are keenly aware of the effect their personal feelings have on the type and quality of health care they are delivering. Teachers can provide students with a forum to discuss these feelings; however, the objective is not to conduct a psychotherapy session. It is possible for the teacher to encourage real expressions of feelings in the group without attempting to intervene in an individual personality conflict. The group experience can provide valuable information to the teacher who may want to help a student understand the need for outside counseling or therapy, but the role of the teacher is to assess whether or not the student has met the objectives of the course.

In addition to being skilled at handling the common problems in groups, the teacher must be able to interpret the themes of the group, that is, those issues that are introduced in one session and reoccur in subsequent group meetings until they are resolved. A small group that is not able to problem solve successfully is a good example. If the students consistently focus their anxiety on those patient-care decisions for which they have sole responsibility, it may be that they need to discuss their fears and fantasies about what would happen if they were to make a mistake. After group members have had an opportunity to discuss and begin resolving a troublesome matter, they are able to move forward in its development.

USING GROUP LEARNING ACTIVITIES

Once the teacher has developed the skills necessary to be an effective teacher in a group, the decisions of when to use what kind of group becomes easier. Often there is no way to determine in advance if a group learning activity will effectively meet certain objectives until it is actually piloted and tried. Again, course objectives and physical limitations often restrict the use of groups within a course. It may be possible to break up a course of 100 students into ten groups with the help of teaching assistants or by the teacher managing the course schedule differently. In other instances, however, this may be neither feasible nor advantageous. Some learning objectives are best accomplished through lecturing to large groups. Groups used incorrectly can be wasteful and frustrating. They are not the answer to all learning or course situations.

Traditionally, clinical supervision for students in the health sciences has been done on a one-to-one basis or in small groups. But another use of the small-group experience is to facilitate the student's learning of content. Learning packages can be used to present content that each student can master independently. Then, small groups can be organized to answer student questions and help students synthesize their new information. This system also provides the teacher with ongoing evaluation of the student's progress toward mastering the objectives of the course.

Teaching content through small-group process involves a role change for both the student and the teacher. For teachers, it requires both a philosophical change and a change of control and responsibility. Teachers must believe that students can learn without them and trust them to do so. They must believe that if students are provided with good learning materials, they will seize the opportunity and learn. Thus, if there are no questions after studying a learning package, the teacher should not assume that the students have not done their work. Instead, the teacher should be pleased and commend the students for their independent learning.

Of course, students are likely to test teachers, particularly during the initiation phase, by not being prepared. Too often, when teaching traditionally, teachers who discover that an outside assignment has not been done by students review the essential points of the assignment, particularly if they are concerned about students being unprepared for clinical situations the next day. If teachers continue to do this in groups, the students quickly perceive that teachers obviously do not mean what they say. As a result, group trust never develops and group growth is at a standstill.

Teachers, when they are being tested, can say, "It was your responsibility to have mastered this content before you came to class. You are responsible for this material and it will not be covered again. We will proceed next week with the new material." In this way, teachers communicate in a very real fashion that students are expected to prepare and master content before the group begins and that they *can* do it.

Once questions are answered, the teacher can then proceed with the group strategy selected to accomplish the objectives and provide an opportunity for problem solving. The teacher has much less control over the problem solving process when a small group is used than when this is done in a large lecture section through calling on students. Once the situation is presented to the students, the teacher needs to allow and encourage the group to problem solve. Even if they seem to be getting off the right track, they must be allowed to continue until one student realizes their error. Students often will ask the teacher if they are correct. They also may finish problem solving and still not realize they have made a mistake. In the latter situation, the teacher needs to correct the students before they leave the group. Usually, however, students realize something is wrong earlier and this experience, while time consuming, helps the students develop a personal awareness of when they have made a mistake. By encouraging students not to use the teacher for answers, the teacher is showing them how to consult and problem solve with each other.

UNIT 3
BIBLIOGRAPHY

Traditional Teaching Strategies

Lecture

EBEL, KENNETH E. *The Craft of Teaching*. San Francisco, Ca.: Jossey Bass, 1976.

    A descriptive treatment of teaching by a master teacher. Discusses the uses and misuses of lecture, as well as other strategies appropriate for college- and university-level teaching. Enjoyable reading.

HYMAN, RONALD T. *Ways of Teaching*. Philadelphia: Lippincott, 1970.

    A thorough analysis of several teaching-learning strategies, discussed for the most part in terms of general education. The section on lecture includes descriptions of the uses of lecture, examples of approaches to lectures, and suggested techniques for organizing and delivering lectures. Recommended reading.

McLEISH, JOHN. *The Lecture Method*. Cambridge, England: Cambridge Institute of Education, 1968.

    A research monograph comprising studies of student retention of lecture material, student attitudes, and how to improve the lecture. Empirical descriptions of the ''spurt-sag-spurt'' phenomenon are informative.

Discussion

GULLEY, HOLBERT E. *Discussion, Conference and Group Process*. 2d ed. New York: Holt, Rinehart and Winston, 1968.

    A basic resource on discussion as a teaching-learning strategy. Combines theoretical and practical approaches to group process with the planning and management of discussion.

HYMAN, RONALD T. *Ways of Teaching*. Philadelphia: Lippincott, 1970.

    Includes a section describing the discussion method; techniques for organizing and conducting discussions with students; the use of the Socratic method as a teaching-learning strategy; and encouraging discovery learning through discussion.

POTTER, DAVID, and MARTIN P. ANDERSEN. *Discussion*. Belmont, Ca.: Wadsworth, 1963.

A readable resource describing practical approaches to discussion as a teaching-learning strategy. Intended to be used as a workbook, it includes suggestions, techniques, and procedures for planning, managing, and evaluating discussion.

Clinical Teaching

COGAN, MORRIS L. *Clinical Supervision*. Boston: Houghton Mifflin, 1973.

Deals with both broad areas of clinical supervisor, e.g., problem areas for clinical supervisors as well as the process of planning clinical experiences. Focuses heavily on the supervisory aspects of clinical teaching. Good reference list at end of book.

SCHWEER, JEAN E., and KRISTINE M. GEBBIE. *Creative Teaching in Clinical Nursing*. St. Louis: C. V. Mosby Co., 1976.

Good comprehensive book on designing and implementing creative teaching approaches to clinical experiences in nursing. Is applicable to all health sciences. Good references and suggested readings at end of each chapter.

WIEDENBACH, ERNESTINE. *Meeting the Realities in Clinical Teaching*. New York: Springer, Inc., 1971.

Uses a prescriptive approach to clinical teaching in nursing, but is applicable to any health science. Contains many useful ideas. Good section on planning and sequencing for clinical experiences.

Laboratory Teaching

POSTLETHWAIT, S. N., J. NOVAK, and H. T. MURRAY, JR. *The Audio-Tutorial Approach to Learning*. 3d ed. Minneapolis: Burgess, 1972.

Does not deal with laboratory teaching per se; rather, discusses principles and procedures of planning and managing the teaching-learning process that facilitate student independence and self-direction. A good reference containing general guidelines for planning and developing unstructured laboratory experiences.

Personalized Instruction

HANAU, LAIA. The Study Game: How to Play and Win with "Statement-Pie." New York: Barnes and Noble Books, 1974.

A resource that can be used with or recommended to students experiencing study-skills difficulties. Although some of the cartoons and narrative might be distracting, the principles and procedures it employs can be highly effective study devices.

HOMME, LLOYD. *How to Use Contingency Contracting in the Classroom*. Champaign, Ill.: Research Press, 1969.

An excellent book that describes the process of contracting with students. The content and approaches described in this book are easily adapted for use with students in the health sciences.

PAUK, WALTER. *How to Study in College*. 2d ed. Boston: Houghton Mifflin, 1974.

Practical discussions directed at students. Presents a variety of basic, supportive, academic, and specialized skills and ways they can be developed. A good resource that can be recommended to students.

ROSENBAUM, PETER S. *Peer-Mediated Instruction.* New York: Teachers College Press, 1973.

A systematic discussion of the development, management, and evaluation of tutoring programs that can be used as adjuncts to formal components of the teaching-learning process. Principles and procedures given are easily applicable to health science education.

RUSSELL, J. D. *Modular Instruction: A Guide to the Design, Selection, Utilization and Evaluation of Modular Materials.* Minneapolis: Burgess, 1974.

Contains information on the background and fundamentals of modular instruction as well as specific procedures for the development of modular materials. Separate chapters cover such topics as defining objectives, analyzing the learner, sequencing modules, and evaluating and using the finished product. Can be used as a reference for designing and managing learning packages, contingency contracting, or tutorials.

Groups

CARTWRIGHT, DARWIN, and ALVIN ZANDER. *Group Dynamics.* 3d ed. New York: Harper & Row, 1968.

The basic resource on groups and group processes. Presents empirical results of research on a variety of aspects of group dynamics. While many papers are technical, all are readable. The best reference for most teacher's questions on groups and group process.

MARRAM, GWEN D. *The Group Approach in Nursing Practice.* St. Louis: C. V. Mosby Co., 1973.

Describes a variety of group situations in which nurses function, such as self-help groups and growth groups. Includes theoretical orientations behind the study and practice of group work.

PFEIFFER, WILLIAM, and JOHN E. JONES. *A Handbook of Structured Experiences for Human Relations Training.* 6 vols. San Diego, Ca.: University Associates, 1973–1977.

Concise, descriptive books of group strategies. The advantage of these books is that the group activities described can be adapted for use in the classroom. A disadvantage is that there is no material on what type of group process might result from using a certain activity. Teachers need to be careful not to use these as cookbooks; rather, they should be regarded as a source of suggested activities.

UNIT 4
THE EVALUATION PROCESS

Evaluation activities provide the means for determining the effectiveness of those activities undertaken in the planning, development, and management stages of teaching. As is true of the other stages, evaluation is not a singular activity, occurring only at the end of a course or unit; rather, it is a dynamic, ongoing activity that contributes to the continued refinement of the teaching-learning process.

It is possible that many teachers, based on past experiences as students or graduate assistants, can begin teaching with some initial ideas about how to approach their teaching responsibilities. It is also possible that they can readily select and develop content for presentation to students, using their expertise in a specific content area to guide their decisions. It is less likely, however, that they will have had personal experience, role models, or formal preparation in planning and conducting evaluation activities. The lack of such preparation frequently leads to evaluation procedures and policies planned and conducted in haphazard fashion, yielding results that are often less than useful or satisfying.

Evaluation is the process of specifying, collecting, and using information for decision making. A variety of decisions concerning the teaching-learning process, made by a variety of individuals, should be based on the information obtained from evaluation activities. Just as the previous stages of teaching are to be approached systematically, so too is the evaluation stage. When conducted systematically, the results of evaluation can be useful and gratifying to teachers, teachers' colleagues, students, and other decision makers.

The purpose of this unit is to introduce teachers to some of the essential principles and techniques of educational evaluation, so that they can begin to develop a systematic approach to evaluation. Chapter 11 describes general principles of evaluation and presents a framework health science teachers might use in approaching evaluation. Chapter 12 describes several common approaches to assessing student learning and suggests ways these approaches can be used to evaluate student achievement of minimal competence and developmental competence objectives. Chapter 13 is concerned with evaluating the teaching-learning process and its parts, while Chapter 14 presents a brief discussion of validity and reliability, two of the major requirements evaluation results must meet if they are to be useful for decision making.

11

PLANNING FOR EVALUATION

Planning and development activities form the foundation for the teaching-learning process, while management activities provide the means for guiding it. Evaluation activities combine to indicate the degree to which the teaching-learning process and its parts have been effective—that is, the degree to which they have contributed to students' achievement of the objectives established for a course.

Teachers in health science programs frequently think of evaluation as the measurement of student achievement, usually through some form of testing procedure. To a lesser extent, they may think of it in terms of student reactions to teaching activities or the process involved in judging professional performance for the purpose of promotion. Also, because evaluation is often thought of as the final step in the sequence of teaching activities, many teachers begin to consider evaluation only when their course or unit is nearing completion. None of these conceptions of evaluation is by itself entirely accurate, nor can any one of them alone determine the effectiveness of the teaching-learning process and its parts.

In more comprehensive terms, evaluation can be viewed as a process of specifying, collecting, and analyzing information for the purpose of decision making (13). It is a systematic, continuous process that begins in the planning stage of an activity and continues through to its conclusion. The results or products of evaluation, the various kinds of information that are collected and analyzed, provide the means for making a variety of decisions, most of which relate to the direction subsequent planning, development, and management activities will take.

SOME GENERAL CHARACTERISTICS OF EVALUATION

The type of educational decisions to be made by a teacher or other individuals connected with the teaching-learning process dictate the type of evaluation activity to be conducted. Evaluation activities are generally of two types: *formative* or *summative* (11). Formative evaluation is concerned with the process of teaching and learning as it occurs, particularly with identifying facets of the process that need to be improved in order to increase effectiveness. Summative evaluation, on the other hand, is concerned with the product or the results of the teaching-learning process; its purpose is to provide some summary or final assessment of the teaching-learning process.

A teacher incorporating a newly developed series of slide-tape programs as an alternate learning approach in a course needs to know how useful and how effective each program is for students using the series on an experimental basis. The results of various evaluation activities will thus be used to make any necessary revisions or modifications in such things as scripts, slides, speed of narration, or continuity of content, so that all the programs in the series can be ready for use on a permanent basis.

The same teacher may also provide students the opportunity to take several self-assessment examinations at different intervals of the course. The purpose of these ungraded examinations is to give students some indication of their progress. The results of the self-assessments can serve to highlight an individual student's need to alter study habits, to concentrate on different content or skill areas, or to continue in the same mode of study.

In both cases the information obtained from evaluation is used for formative decision making; that is, decisions that result in modification or revision of the teaching-learning process in order to improve it, as well as retention of those features that are found satisfactory.

Summative evaluation activities are conducted to obtain information pertinent to final decisions about the product or result of the teaching-learning process. These decisions can range from determining the overall effectiveness of the process in promoting student learning to determining final levels of student performance. They assume that appropriate decisions have already been made and acted on as a result of formative evaluation activities, so that the teaching-learning process has proceeded as effectively and efficiently as possible.

The teacher in the previous example may ask students, colleagues, and practitioners to assess the slide-tape series as a learning tool, once any necessary revisions have been made and it has been included as a part of the course. The results of their assessments would contribute to a summary decision of the effectiveness of the series and thus would determine whether or not the series should continue to be used.

As the course progresses, the teacher conducts several evaluation activities to assess students' performance. These activities can include such things as laboratory projects, papers, clinical simulation exercises, or problem-solving examinations. The results of these assessments, when taken together, provide the basis for determining each student's level of performance in the course and thus the basis for pass/fail or final grade decisions.

In these instances, the evaluation information obtained is used to make summative decisions; that is, decisions that reflect a final judgment of the worth or effectiveness of some facet of the teaching-learning process.

Just as information needs for different kinds of decisions dictate the purpose and the type of evaluation activity conducted—either formative or summative—so too do they have a bearing on the manner in which an evaluation activity is carried out. To be useful and to meet the specific needs for which it was intended, any evaluation activity must be conducted so that *appropriate* and *repeatable* information is obtained.

A physical therapist working with a recent amputee and an immunologist studying chronic granulomatous disease in a research laboratory function in different environments, with different purposes guiding their efforts. Both must be concerned, however, that the kinds of techniques, procedures, or methods they employ are appropriate, so that the results they finally obtain come as close as possible to fulfilling their original purposes. Further, both must be concerned that the techniques, procedures, or methods they use will ensure that the same results can be obtained on other occasions—i.e., the physical therapist's methods will assist similar amputee patients in regaining mobility; the immunologist's laboratory procedures will produce the same results each time a specific experiment is repeated.

The physical therapist and immunologist, as well as any other health care professional, can transfer the kinds of considerations guiding their professional activities to their educational activities. Just as they must be able to establish the appropriateness and repeatability of the results they obtain in the clinic or laboratory, so too must they be able to establish the appropriateness and repeatability of evaluation results obtained in the classroom. Clinicians and researchers generally find that the requirements of both settings can be satisfied in similar ways and that the process becomes much easier to accomplish in the classroom as more practical experience is gained.

Appropriateness of educational evaluation is generally discussed in terms of the *validity* of evaluation results, the extent to which results obtained from any evaluation activity serve the purpose for which they were intended (5). If an evaluation device, such as a simulation exercise or media evaluation form, measures the precise characteristics it was designed to measure, valid results will be obtained. In addition, because validity is a characteristic specific to a particular use or purpose, it is considered a matter of degree rather than an all-or-none proposition (4). A multiple-choice midterm exam in anatomy, for example, could have a high degree of validity for indicating students' performance in the first half of the course, a moderate degree of validity for predicting their performance in the second half of the course, and no validity for predicting their performance in biochemistry.

A teacher's primary concern in developing any evaluation activity, then, is ensuring that it is valid (appropriate) for a particular purpose, so that it produces valid results. Specific approaches to establishing the validity of various educational evaluation activities are discussed in subsequent chapters.

Repeatability in educational evaluation is generally discussed in terms of the *reliability* of evaluation results, the extent to which results obtained from any evaluation activity are stable or consistent, or can be generalized from one group or situation to a similar one (12). Like validity, reliability is directly related to the intended purpose of an evaluation activity. The results of a test intended to measure students' mastery of minimal competence objectives would probably demonstrate satisfactory reliability when obtained on two different occasions from the same or similar groups of students (e.g., a test-retest measure of reliability). Results of the same test would demonstrate insufficient reliability, however, if analyzed according to procedures normally used for achievement tests intended to discriminate among students. This discrepancy occurs because, unlike validity, reliability is entirely a statistical property of evaluation results. Methods for computing reliability must therefore be selected in light of the purpose of the evaluation activity. Several of these methods are presented in the following chapters.

An evaluation activity can yield highly reliable but invalid results. Such a situation may occur, for example, when an achievement test originally intended to assess students' problem-solving abilities in fact measures only their ability to recall specific pieces of information. This situation would provide the teacher with consistent, repeatable measures of the wrong thing; thus, the information would be essentially unusable.

An evaluation activity can also yield highly unreliable results. This frequently occurs with many teachers' evaluation activities, because of some problem in their construction or administration. It can also occur because of some chance fluctuation in student characteristics, such as fatigue or emotional strain, or because the characteristics being measured are themselves unstable, such as student attitudes toward an emotion-charged issue. In any of these situations, validity is decreased markedly, for the original purpose of evaluation cannot be fulfilled by unreliable results.

Validity and reliability are two of the most important conditions to be satisfied in any evaluation activity; they are also two that are often overlooked or undervalued. Teachers who take time to ensure that these conditions are met also ensure that the evaluation information they obtain will be useful for later decision making.

THE EVALUATION PROCESS

The validity and reliability of evaluation activities are greatly enhanced if a systematic approach to their planning and implementation is followed. A systematic approach assumes that preparation for evaluation is an integral part of the planning stage of teaching, rather than an unwanted task postponed as long as possible. It also assumes that the results of evaluation contribute to the direction later planning, development, and management activities take.

The systematic nature of the educational evaluation process is analogous to the systematic process involved in conducting a patient assessment. In the patient assessment, the steps or procedures of an *examination* are requisite to establishing a *diagnosis,* while a carefully developed diagnosis allows some *prescription* for care to be made.

Throughout the patient-assessment process, information of different kinds (physical, emotional, social) must be collected and analyzed to yield a diagnosis. The information can be derived from different sources (patient, patient's past health history, patient's family or friends) and by different individuals (physician, nurse, physician's assistant), often over a period of time (e.g., the time required to confirm the presence of a collagen disease). The collected data are analyzed in terms of criteria appropriate to specific states found on a wellness-illness continuum, leading to the formulation of a diagnosis of the patient's current status. The diagnosis then provides the basis for prescribing a specific regimen of care.

Several characteristics of the patient-assessment process are directly applicable to the educational evaluation process. Once the purposes of a course or unit have been defined in terms of specific learning objectives, the evaluation components constituting the examination phase can be planned. Just as health professionals planning a patient assessment know the type of information they will be seeking and how they intend to obtain it, so, too, must teachers identify information needed for educational decision making, the sources most able to provide that information, the criteria with which to later judge the information, and the methods for collecting it. These activities are all requisite to collecting evaluation information.

When the activities of the examination phase have been completed, those of the diagnostic phase can take place. Here teachers analyze the evaluation information they obtained and interpret the results of the analysis, so that some conclusions can be reached about the teaching-learning process or its parts.

The diagnosis phase, involving the analysis and interpretation of evaluation information, provides the basis for the prescription phase, wherein those in decision making positions place value judgments on what has been accomplished and recommend appropriate action to be taken in response to the evaluation results. A graphic summary of the evaluation process is given in Fig. 11.1.

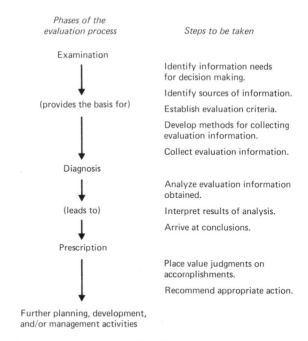

Fig. 11.1
Summary of the evaluation process.

Examination

The Examination Phase

Identify information needs for decision making.
Identify sources of evaluation information.
Establish criteria for evaluation.
Develop methods for collecting evaluation information.
Collect evaluation information.

Identify information needs for decision making   The essential first step in the evaluation process is identifying individuals or groups of individuals who need to receive evaluation information from the teacher, as well as the types of information each requires for decision making. Proceeding through this identification process not only contributes to the orderly, systematic nature of evaluation activities, it also greatly reduces the possibility that a teacher, after concluding teaching activities, will be asked to provide evaluation information that is no longer available for collection. Many teachers have found themselves in this awkward position because, through inexperience or insufficient communication, they considered only short-term or personal evaluation needs.

Teachers can begin the identification process with an examination of their own needs, but they must be sure to branch out from there. The most obvious and most important evaluation information need of teachers involves *student performance* in a course or unit of instruction. Information describing student performance permits teachers to make pass/fail or achieved/not achieved decisions about their students as they progress through the course; it also permits them to ultimately assign some grade, a form of value judgment, to each student's performance upon completion of a course or unit.

Students also require information regarding their performance. They need to know whether or not they are satisfactorily meeting the learning objectives established. This information is most useful if mechanisms for periodic feedback from the teacher are incorporated in the course (6), such as a series of self-assessment examinations or written assignments or projects. Further, if alternative learning activities are available, students also need to know which alternatives will assist them in learning most effectively and efficiently. Thus, information obtained from pretests, from learning-style or cognitive-style inventories, and from student performance in various learning activities should be shared with students.

Information concerning student performance can be useful for other individuals or committees within the school or department. A teacher's assessment of student performance provides the basis for decisions regarding individual student's progression from one course or level of courses to another. Such decisions usually entail approving a student's promotion in a curriculum; they can also entail suggesting remedial or enrichment work for specific students, requiring that a particular course or unit be repeated, or recommending that a student be dropped from the educational program. Whichever of these decisions is to be made, those who finalize the decision must have information describing student performance that is as accurate and extensive as possible. A single grade reflecting performance on a final examination, for example, contributes little useful information for deciding exactly why a particular student is experiencing learning difficulties.

Student-performance information often is needed by promotions or budget committees. In those institutions where teaching is a valued activity, the extent to which students achieve course objectives can comprise one indicator of a teacher's effectiveness and can be considered when decisions are made regarding merit raises or promotions. Further, student-performance information can also be useful for budget committees charged with deciding, for example, whether or not to continue funding a teacher's media development activities or whether or not to provide funding for further educational innovations planned by a department or division. In these instances, information about the performance of students using alternate materials or resources can be included with information describing the financial outlay associated with them.

Teachers almost always need evaluation information concerning the *material resources* used in a course or unit. Obtaining feedback about the relative effectiveness, utility, or efficiency of the various materials used in the teaching-learning process provides one source of information for later decisions in the areas of planning, development, and management (7). Discovering inconsistencies or inaccuracies in a course syllabus can lead to appropriate revisions; determining that a series of slide-tape programs was a highly effective learning tool can help to confirm its use as an alternate strategy in subsequent offerings of the course. In these and other instances, evaluation information can establish a valid base for a teacher's educational decision making.

A teacher's colleagues may also require information obtained from the evaluation of material resources. Other teachers in the same department may be interested in using one or more of a teacher's mediated materials in their own teaching or may be interested in developing their own. In either case, information about the relative effectiveness and efficiency of such materials will be useful to them. A teacher's department chairman or the members of a budget committee may also be interested in examining effectiveness and efficiency information; for example, they may want to know the financial commitment required to plan and produce the videotapes used in an introductory physiology course, how well students were able to perform later as a result of viewing the tapes, and any savings realized in instructor or laboratory-assistant time. By extension, these kinds of information would also be quite useful for colleagues teaching in other institutions who are considering purchasing copies of a teacher's materials or developing their own.

Teachers need evaluation information about the *activities of the teaching-learning process* in the same way they need information describing material resources. Decisions to retain or discontinue specific activities, such as guest-lecture presentations, role-playing sequences, or simulation exercises, cannot legitimately be made on the basis of a teacher's intuition or feelings. Further, if a teacher is earnest in providing as many alternative teaching-learning experiences as is practicable in order to meet student needs and interests, then evaluation information regarding the degree of "fit" between specific experiences and specific types of students is essential.

A teacher's colleagues are often interested in the evaluation results of specific activities. A colleague who is considering the inclusion of simulation exercises may want to know how effective similar exercises have been in other courses. Another may need to know how different types of students have reacted to specific strategies—for example, how borderline-ability students have responded to role playing in another course. Finally, a teacher's colleagues sitting on promotions committees are likely to be interested in various types of evaluation information as one indicator of the teacher's effectiveness.

Evaluation information describing a *teacher's own contribution to the teaching-learning process* is sought by those teachers committed to professional growth. The process of discovering one's strengths and weaknesses in such activities as the delivery of a lecture, the organization of laboratory experiences, or the guidance of seminar-discussion sessions is not, however, accomplished in one semester. Nor is it accomplished by teachers acting alone, reflecting on their own performance. Information obtained from peers, students, and self on an ongoing basis can greatly assist one's professional development. By extension, any improvement in a teacher's contribution to the teaching-learning process almost always enhances student learning.

Identify sources of evaluation information   When teachers have identified the kinds of evaluation information they need, either immediately or eventually, and have located any other individuals or groups who also require this information for their decision making, the next step is to select the sources of the evaluation information. Just as teachers must be concerned with gathering a variety of kinds of evaluation information to provide the most comprehensive feedback possible, so too must they be concerned with obtaining that information from a variety of sources. The basic guideline for this step is to identify all those individuals who are in the best positions to provide specific types of information.

Because of their intimate involvement in the teaching-learning process, *students* are in the best position to provide evaluative information about many facets of the process. Their performance on paper-and-pencil examinations, simulation exercises, projects, or clinical assignments indicates the extent to which they are achieving course or unit objectives. By extension, their performance can also indicate the teacher's effectiveness or the effectiveness of resource materials or learning activities. If given the opportunity to respond to appropriate questions or criteria, students are able to provide valid, reliable, and usable evaluation information (3). They can indicate how useful they find the organization and sequence of activities in a course, the material resources, and the personal contributions of the teacher to the teaching-learning process. They are far less able and qualified, however, to evaluate such factors as the appropriateness of content selected or the professional competence of their teachers.

A teacher's *colleagues* can be the best source of evaluation information dealing with most aspects of the teaching-learning process. Fellow teachers, as content experts and health care professionals themselves, can provide information that both complements and supplements that supplied by students. They can be asked to evaluate factors as diverse as the appropriateness of materials and methods selected for use in a course; the effectiveness of the teacher in managing classroom, clinical, or laboratory activities; the performance of students in settings outside the teacher's classroom; and the contribution that the course and the teacher make to achieving the general purposes of the educational program.

In situations where colleague evaluation is the exception rather than the rule, experienced teachers interested in peer review may feel more comfortable than junior faculty in soliciting such evaluation. They may also feel more competent in knowing which colleagues possess the expertise to evaluate different facets of the teaching-learning process. New teachers, on the other hand, may be reluctant to seek out colleagues for evaluation purposes shortly after assuming their teaching responsibilities. Depending on institutional requirements, their best course of action may be to spend a semester getting to know their fellow teachers professionally, in the classroom, clinic, or laboratory, with one end in view: to discover who may be most willing and able to provide evaluation information.

Local health-care practitioners can be fruitful sources of evaluation information for several facets of the teaching-learning process. Practitioners serving in a preceptor role are able to evaluate student performance in a practical, working environment. This kind of information can be used by the teacher to supplement in-class performance evaluation or to add a type of predictive quality to in-class performance measures. Practitioners are also able to indicate the relevance of educational materials, resources, and sometimes methods to the practice environment, as well as to comment on the appropriateness of course or resource content to practice. A nursing supervisor in a convalescent home, for example, should be able to provide very useful reactions to slide-tape programs dealing with care of the geriatric cancer patient. This information would be useful in developing educational experiences for a nursing assistant's program.

Teachers themselves are sources of evaluation information. They must evaluate student performance, such as clinical, group, or laboratory work, that is not amenable to paper-and-pencil assessment. They might also record their reactions to specific materials or strategies used in the teaching-learning process. While it may be difficult for teachers who have spent a great deal of their time developing media resources to evaluate objectively their utility as learning experiences, their attempts at critical appraisals can be used to supplement student, colleague, or practitioner evaluations.

In settings where sufficient equipment and appropriate consultative personnel are available, teachers may also evaluate their own teaching performance through some form of microteaching, in which a segment or series of segments of their in-class performance is videotaped for later analysis with a teaching consultant (9). Like other types of evaluation information, the purpose of microteaching is to obtain data that will contribute to the improvement of the teacher's performance and, consequently, to the enhancement of student learning.

A graphic summary of the types of information different sources can provide to meet different evaluation information needs is depicted in Table 11.1. These types of information are discussed in subsequent chapters.

Establish criteria for evaluation   Criteria for specific evaluation activities are established before any evaluation takes place. By deciding on evaluation criteria

Table 11.1.
Most Common Types of Evaluation Information Provided by Sources to Meet Information Needs

SOURCES OF INFORMATION	INFORMATION NEEDS			
	Student Learning	Material Resources	Teaching-Learning Activities	Teacher Contributions
Students	Performance information from internally constructed examinations, projects, etc. and from externally constructed examinations—e.g., National Board examinations.	Performance information; reactions to resources; participation in experimental studies.	Participation in experimental studies; reaction to specific activities, strategies, etc.	Reaction to contributions to individual learning.
Teachers	Observation of in-class, clinical, and laboratory performance; problem-solving skills.	Observation of student use. Professional opinions: relevance to needs, purposes, objectives; costs, cost benefits	Observation.	Self-analysis through microteaching or similar procedures.
Teacher's Colleagues	Observation of performance in scheduled activities.	Professional opinions: relevance to educational needs, principles, objectives; costs, cost benefits.	Observation.	Observation; inferences drawn from student performance.
Practitioners	Observation of performance in practical environments.	Professional opinions: relevance to practice, objectives.	Observation.	Observation; inferences drawn from student performance.

during the planning stage of instruction, teachers implicitly contribute to the consistency and validity of all activities of the teaching-learning process. Further, they avoid the common experience of arbitrarily arriving at some criteria after evaluation results are in and require interpretation.

Criteria for evaluating student performance are developed as extensions of the objectives and learning activities of a course or unit. Minimal competence objectives and their associated learning activities represent knowledge or skills that are basic or prerequisite to later course work or to developmental knowledge or skills. Thus, a teacher would expect all students to demonstrate a high level of proficiency in meeting these objectives (8). Developmental competence objectives and their associated learning activities represent knowledge or skills that each student is encouraged to pursue to the best of personal abilities. Because of inherent differences in student abilities, teachers would expect students to demonstrate different levels of proficiency in meeting these objectives (2) and would establish performance criteria accordingly. Specific techniques for establishing criteria for minimal and developmental competence objectives are discussed in Chapter 13.

The major criteria for evaluating material resources are derived from the learning objectives students are to accomplish through their use. Usually such resources as slide-tapes, videotapes, or printed handouts are developed or purchased to assist students in accomplishing specific minimal competence objectives. The major criteria for their evaluation then becomes the extent to which all students demonstrate a high level of proficiency on the objectives following use of the resource.

Additional criteria for evaluating material resources relate to their efficiency. Teachers incorporating any new or additional resources in their teaching activities are usually expected to show that factors such as cost of production or procurement; time commitment of faculty, faculty assistants, or students; or amortization and depreciation make the resource at least as efficient in the long run as a traditional method, its positive effect on student learning notwithstanding (7).

Teachers planning to incorporate new material resources in their course or unit, either by adding them to the set of available learning activities or by using them as replacements for existing materials or methods, should be concerned in the planning stage of instruction with establishing both effectiveness and efficiency criteria for their later evaluation. Techniques for developing these kinds of criteria are discussed in Chapter 14.

Criteria for evaluating the teaching-learning process, its parts, and the teacher's contributions to it are derived from the learning objectives of a course. The major criteria for evaluating each of these aspects are the extent to which they are both appropriate and effective in assisting students achieve specific objectives. In addition, the criteria reflect such factors as the nature of the students being taught, the situation or setting in which the teaching-learning process occurs, and the resources and constraints affecting the manner in which the process takes place.

Regardless of what is to be evaluated, teachers must be certain that criteria for evaluation are established as specific activities are planned and developed. This not only enhances the consistency and coherence of the teaching-learning process, it also provides the means for prompt, efficient interpretation of evaluation results, so that appropriate decision making can take place.

Develop methods for collecting evaluation information   Methods for collecting evaluation information are planned and developed before the teaching-learning process begins. To do otherwise is to diminish the validity and the consistency of the process as a whole. A common practice of many teachers is to construct achievement examinations or other evaluation mechanisms shortly before the day students are to respond to them. This practice reduces the possibility that all appropriate factors will be evaluated and that specific evaluation activities will contribute to improving the teaching-learning process.

In planning and developing methods for collecting evaluation information, teachers consider in tandem the overall goals of their course, their specific learning objectives, the types and sources of evaluation information they need to collect, and the resources and constraints they have already identified as having some effect on the teaching-learning process.

The goals and objectives of a course or unit provide the foundation for explicit criteria for any evaluation activity. Teachers therefore decide which methods of assessment are likely to obtain the most useful information for comparing specific factors with preestablished criteria. Direct observation of student performance, for example, may provide better information than a multiple-choice examination when student achievement of developmental competence objectives is to be assessed, while a short multiple-choice test may be put to better use in evaluating the contribution a slide-tape program makes to student achievement of specific minimal competence objectives. Further, because of the variable nature of human performance, both of students and teachers, and because of the error problem associated with most measurement or evaluation devices (1), single attempts at evaluation seldom provide adequate information about most facets of the teaching-learning process. Teachers must therefore also consider which combination of methods or devices will ensure the collection of adequate evaluation information. Various methods and devices are discussed in Chapters 13 and 14.

A teacher's choice of specific approaches to collecting evaluation information should lead to the most effective and efficient methods available for comparing the obtained information with the criteria that have already been established. Evaluating each student's achievement of both minimal and developmental competence objectives, for example, requires different analytic procedures than does evaluating the effectiveness of a slide-tape program in terms of the percentage of students who meet the established performance level of a multiple-choice quiz.

A useful method for determining which specific devices or procedures to use in later analyses entails the construction of mock tables and reporting mechanisms similar to those that will eventually be used to record the evaluation information. Once teachers can visualize the final arrangement of evaluation information needed, it becomes easier to work backward through the analysis process to the selection of analysis methods. This approach is not unlike that used in conducting a research project. Before research investigation begins, the researcher organizes data tables and reporting mechanisms which will later contain the data obtained to test hypotheses or answer questions posed in the research. Such preparation serves not only to further organize the researcher's thinking, it also contributes to selecting or confirming the choice of data-analysis methods—for example, data tables can indicate the need for the proper form of statistical technique to test research hypotheses.

Closely associated with the choice of specific analysis procedures is the teacher's need to confirm the availability of time, financial, and personnel resources for information analysis. Many schools, divisions, or departments provide some form of support for faculty to process the analysis of evaluation information. This support can range from the services provided by a central resource group of evaluation consultants, to the availability of faculty assistants or clerical help, to financial assistance for machine processing of the information. The extent to which these resources are available necessarily influences the specific analytic methods and procedures a teacher can select.

Collect evaluation information   The actual process of collecting evaluation information completes the examination phase of educational evaluation. If a systematic approach has been taken to planning and conducting the previous activities, the evaluation information collected will provide a legitimate basis for eventual decision making.

Evaluation information can be collected in many ways, depending on the teacher's purposes. Possibilities include achievement testing, observing student performance, distributing course/instructor evaluations, or requesting colleagues to evaluate a series of learning packages. The process of obtaining information using any collection method is affected by the nature of the assessment technique employed and by its relative obtrusiveness on the teaching-learning process.

The assessment technique chosen depends on the specific type of evaluation information to be collected. A problem-solving exercise simulating an actual patient case history, for example, may be most appropriate for assessing students' approaches to particular developmental competence objectives. Such an exercise may necessitate the preparation of written programmed materials, videotapes, and worksheets for collecting student responses. It also requires that students be familiar with the technique before using it, that sufficient time be allowed for students to complete the exercise, and that procedures be established for providing feedback to students as soon after the assessment session as possible. These characteristics and requirements combine to indicate how the exercise is to be arranged for, administered, and completed.

If evaluation is seen as a natural part of the teaching-learning process, the collection of information using any evaluation technique can occur unobtrusively. Oftentimes the act of evaluating influences the subjects being evaluated; for example, students in a clinical setting who know their performance is being observed and rated are likely to experience some increased anxiety. Increased anxiety here can have a negative effect on their performance. Similarly, student course-evaluation forms distributed by disinterested teachers are often viewed skeptically by students as a waste of time. This attitude necessarily colors any responses they might give. If teachers begin their courses or units with an explanation of evaluation policies, activities, and criteria and present evaluation as an integral part of the teaching-learning process, they are likely to find that the eventual collection of information does not obtrude on the teaching-learning process. Thus, they are more able to collect valid, usable evaluation data.

Diagnosis

The Diagnosis Phase

Analyze evaluation information obtained.
Interpret results of analysis.

Analyze evaluation information obtained   After evaluation information is collected, it is analyzed to allow the teacher and any other user of the information to begin decision making. Analysis usually entails reorganizing the obtained raw data to make it amenable to interpretation. The analysis of a student's numerical responses to a simulation exercise might result in something like the following: "Taylor made 9 out of 13 correct decisions in the first decision sequence of the exercise, yielding a Diagnostic Index of 14/18, accompanied by the following rationale. . . ." The analysis of student responses to a course/instructor evaluation form might be done by computer according to sections of the evaluation form (e.g., "Course Content," "Learning Activities") and restated in terms of the mean response and its standard deviation for each question or statement. In either case, "raw data" or information in an essentially unusable form is reorganized and presented in a form ready for interpretation.

The selection of procedures to analyze evaluation information is completed in the examination phase of evaluation and depends on the type of evaluation technique chosen to collect information. A multiple-choice, self-assessment examination, for example, is analyzed differently from the comments provided by a group of teachers evaluating a colleague's teaching. Procedure selection also depends on availability of resources; most often selection becomes a matter of choosing between manual or automated analysis. A teacher constructing a simulation exercise in a department where no other simulations are used has to rely on manual scoring to analyze student responses. The same teacher, on the other hand, may be able to send student responses to a course/instructor evaluation form to a central data-processing center for tabulation and analysis.

Interpret the results of evaluation   The interpretation of evaluation results entails comparing analyzed information with criteria in order to arrive at some conclusion about the activity evaluated.

The objectivity of interpretation can vary depending on the type of criteria being used. One teacher may simply have some general criteria in mind when grading student responses to an essay examination; another may grade student responses according to a points system developed for ideal answers to each question. The latter procedure almost always results in more objective interpretation of results and allows more appropriate conclusions to be drawn about each student's work.

Accurate interpretation of evaluation results requires teachers to have a good working knowledge of the information collection and analysis methods they employ. A teacher incorporating the use of *a priori* performance standards for a multiple-choice test, for example, must be thoroughly familiar with scoring and analysis procedures if the test is to have any value as an assessment device. Likewise, a teacher using multipoint rating scales to obtain students' responses to course/instructor evaluations must know what a standard deviation is and what it means in order to interpret the results of an analysis of student responses.

The interpretation of evaluation results often requires attention to factors that might normally seem extraneous. Students' evaluation of a particular teacher's course may be consistently positive, but the same teacher may get negative results when evaluated for contributions made to a team-taught clinical rotation. An examination of information obtained from sources other than current student evaluations may indicate this teacher's clinical setting has been negatively evaluated in the past, primarily because scheduling problems caused more students to be assigned to it than could reasonably be accommodated. In this instance, if additional information had not been sought, an interpretation of the teacher's clinical evaluation results might have led to the unwarranted conclusion that the teacher's clinical performance was deficient, rather than to the conclusion that a long-term problem exists in scheduling procedures.

If the steps taken in the examination and diagnosis phases are approached systematically, evaluation results will undoubtedly be valid and reliable and will allow for proper interpretation and accurate conclusions. As is the case in medical decision making, proper conclusions can be reached at the end of a diagnosis provided the actions leading to it are well conceived, objective, and systematically carried through.

Prescription

The Prescription Phase
Place value judgments on accomplishments. Recommend appropriate action.

Place value judgments on accomplishments   A value judgment is an expression of a preference or an estimation of the general worth of some thing, arrived at by comparisons with an accepted standard. In the teaching-learning process, it represents a decision that the object of judgment contributes positively or negatively to fulfilling the purposes of teaching and learning. A media resource, a teacher's lectures, or a laboratory experience is judged as contributing or not contributing to the preparation of health care professionals, the central, valued purpose of anyone connected with the teaching-learning process in the health sciences.

Standards for arriving at value judgments are derived as the general planning process takes place. They stem from the overall goals of an educational program and from the learning objectives of a course or unit. Because of their importance to the evaluation process, standards, the rationale for choosing them, and the persons or material to be judged by them must be agreed on and made known before the conduct of any evaluation activity (10); otherwise, judgments eventually rendered are likely to be fragmented and of questionable validity.

Individuals in decision-making roles, whether students, teachers, peers, or others, are continually called on to make value judgments as a result of evaluation activities. Students judge their passing scores on mastery tests as "good," for these test results indicate they have met specific objectives that form a part of their professional preparation. Students' negative evaluations of a teacher's lectures are judged by the teacher as "unsatisfactory," for skill in lecturing is necessary when teaching a group of 130 students. A media-resources committee judges a second-year teacher's slide-tape programs as "excellent," for the well-constructed programs represent a first step toward the development of learning packages.

Each of these judgments would be made by comparing the results of some evaluation activity with standards reflecting the overall purposes of the education program. Without such standards having been established and articulated, however, the same students might have viewed passing scores as good simply because passing scores are valued for their own sake; the teacher might have interpreted negative lecture evaluations as unsatisfactory because other members of the department are considered good lecturers; the media-resources committee might have looked favorably at the new teacher's media development activities only because no other faculty members have shown an interest in expanding media use. Such judgments bear little relationship to the objectives of the teaching-learning process and the overall purposes of the educational program. It is therefore important for teachers to take a systematic approach to planning the teaching-learning process and to planning and conducting evaluation activities, for such an approach necessarily generates the standards by which value judgments are eventually made.

Recommend appropriate action   The final step in the evaluation process consists of recommending some action to be taken on the basis of judgments made. If evaluation standards, procedures, and results are valid, then the resultant judgments will be valid also and will lead to the recommendation of appropriate action.

Recommendation of some action represents a transitional step in the evaluation process, for while any action taken is itself an end point, it is also a starting point for further activities. Thus, a teacher's recommendation that students proceed to the next unit of study is based on the results of a series of teaching, learning, and evaluation activities, which led to the judgment that students had completed work necessary for achieving specific learning objectives. The teacher's action also forms the basis for subsequent activities, such as arranging for the next unit's clinical learning experiences, coordinating students' use of learning packages, and scheduling and conducting a series of performance observations.

Any action recommended as the result of evaluation activities shares this transitional quality; it reflects the cyclic, interrelated nature of a teacher's planning, development, management, and evaluation activities.

REFERENCES

1. CRONBACK, LEE J. *Essentials of Psychological Testing.* 3d ed. New York: Harper & Row, 1970.
2. EBEL, ROBERT L. *Measuring Educational Achievement.* Englewood Cliffs, N.J.: Prentice-Hall, 1965.
3. EBLE, KENNETH G. *Professors as Teachers.* San Francisco, Ca.: Jossey-Bass, 1972.
4. GRONLUND, NORMAN E. *Measurement and Evaluation in Teaching.* 2d ed. New York: Macmillan, 1971.
5. KERLINGER, FRED N. *Foundations of Behavioral Research.* 2d ed. New York: Holt, Rinehart and Winston, 1973.
6. KULHANY, RAYMOND W. "Feedback in Written Instruction." *Review of Educational Research* 47 (1977): 211–232.
7. LAWSON, TOM E. *Formative Instructional Product Evaluation.* Englewood Cliffs, N.J.: Educational Technology Publications, 1974.

8. MILLMAN, JASON. "Passing Scores and Test Lengths for Domain-Referenced Measures." *Review of Educational Research* 43 (1973): 205–215.

9. OLIVERO, JAMES L. *Micro-Teaching: Medium for Improving Instruction.* Columbus, Ohio: Merrill, 1970.

10. PROVUS, MALCOLM. *Discrepancy Evaluation.* Berkeley, Ca.: McCutchan, 1971.

11. SCRIVEN, MICHAEL. "The Methodology of Evaluation." In *Perspectives of Curriculum Evaluation* (AERA Monograph Series on Curriculum Evaluation, No. 1.). Chicago: Rand McNally, 1967, pp. 39–83.

12. STANLEY, JULIAN C. "Reliability." In Robert L. Thorndike, ed. *Educational Measurement.* 2d ed. Washington, D.C.: American Council on Education, 1971, pp. 356–442.

13. STUFFLEBEAM, DANIEL L. et al. *Educational Evaluation and Decision Making.* Itasca, Ill.: Peacock, 1971.

12
ASSESSING STUDENT LEARNING

The primary educational responsibility of health science teachers is to guide students through a professional preparation program. Thus, the assessment of student learning is their foremost evaluation activity. Its results represent professional acknowledgement that students have accomplished one segment or series of segments leading to a professional degree.

The assessment of student learning can take place in a variety of forms, under a variety of conditions, and at a variety of times during a course or unit of study. The exact nature of this assessment is defined as teachers plan the teaching-learning process. As discussed earlier, a teacher's plans necessarily reflect the unique character of a course's specific objectives, subject content, students, and environmental resources and constraints. Thus, it naturally follows that plans for assessing student learning must reflect these same idiosyncracies. Hence, the evaluation techniques selected by one teacher may be inappropriate or infeasible for another. One teacher may develop simulation exercises, mediated self-assessment examinations, and a final essay examination, while another may be unable to use any of these devices in a survey course of 300 students. Teachers should become familiar with a variety of approaches to assessing student learning in order to make knowledgeable selections that best meet their evaluation information needs.

GENERAL CRITERIA FOR ASSESSING STUDENT LEARNING

The assessment of student learning has tended to follow a common pattern in many health science courses: a test is developed, generally multiple-choice, intended to represent the material "covered" in a course or unit; then, the test is administered to a group of students whose composite results form the criteria for assigning grades.

This approach has its merits and may be appropriate in instances where discrimination among students' performance forms the basis for placement, selection, or similar decisions—e.g., an annual examination administered by a state licensing agency. As a general assessment approach, however, it fails to deal adequately with many of the issues discussed in previous chapters, among them the use of differing levels or types of objectives, the recognition of the individuality of students, and the provision of alternative learning experiences in a course or unit.

An alternate approach that permits a variety of educational issues to be addressed and applies to a variety of assessment purposes and procedures places the establishment of criteria at the beginning of the assessment process rather than at the end. The basis for the approach is found in the use of minimal and developmental competence learning objectives. By incorporating this system of objectives in the teaching-learning process, the teacher explicitly acknowledges the different types or levels of content, skills, or abilities they represent and implicitly acknowledges the different types of assessment and grading they suggest. Each of these factors has an influence on the development of criteria for assessing student learning, as well as on the process for developing tests or other assessment devices.

Minimal Competence and Developmental Competence Objectives

Minimal competence objectives can provide direction for confronting subject content or information of a finite nature (e.g., "Describe the structure of the hexose monophosphate shunt"); they can represent approaches to common conventions or procedures (e.g., "Outline Frenkel's exercises for tabetic ataxia"); or they can indicate that basic skills are expected to be performed (e.g., "Start a superficial forearm vein Butterfly IV"). In essence, minimal competence objectives represent material that can be characterized as finite, basic, or essential for public safety; that can be expected to be mastered by all students; and that is requisite to students' developmental capabilities and to their approaches to developmental competence objectives.

Developmental competence objectives represent abilities that students are expected to develop according to their own individual capabilities. In general, they indicate approaches to such behaviors and abilities as problem solving, conceptualizing, or valuing, abilities that students are expected to develop to differing degrees (e.g., "Citing appropriate tests and studies, develop a differential diagnosis to distinguish between rheumatoid arthritis and systemic lupus erythematosus").

While indicating behaviors that are considerably broader in scope than those represented by minimal competence objectives, developmental competence objectives are individualistic in that their achievement depends on each student's unique cognitive abilities and the pace or manner in which these abilities are developed. Because the two types of objectives represent different approaches to subject content and student behaviors, they require assessment techniques that recognize these differences.

The teacher's purpose in assessing students' achievement of minimal competence objectives is to determine whether or not each student has learned specific subject content or can perform specific skills. Objective-based techniques, such as multiple-choice tests or checklist skills examinations, may thus be most appropriate and convenient for the teacher's purpose and for the type of content or skills considered (6). Such nonobjective techniques as short-answer essays, projects, or report papers could also be constructed to assess student achievement of minimal competence objectives.

The teacher's purpose in assessing students' achievement of developmental competence objectives is to determine the students' approaches to the objectives, as well as the degree to which the objectives have been attained. Unlike minimal competence objectives, which are meant to be mastered by all students, developmental competence objectives are expected to be pursued to differing degrees. They therefore require assessment formats that allow particular abilities, such as problem solving, to be displayed by students. Subjective-based techniques, like performance observation, essay examinations, oral examinations, or projects, are usually most appropriate for meeting the purposes of this type of assessment (6). Simulation exercises and well-constructed multiple-choice examinations can also be effective measures.

The assignment of grades or similar value judgments to student performance on tests is directly affected by the type of objectives being measured. In its simplest terms, the judgment of students' achievement of minimal competence objectives represents a yes/no or pass/fail decision; students either have achieved specific objectives or they have not. Grading concepts associated with mastery learning are appropriate here, as are those associated with criterion-referenced measurement (5), for all students are expected to demonstrate mastery or to meet successfully the criteria represented by the objectives.

The grading or judging of student achievement of developmental competence objectives must reflect the nature of the objectives and the nature of the students being assessed. The same standards or criteria used for minimal competence objectives are therefore inappropriate, since student performance on these objectives cannot be judged in absolute terms. Rather, individual student performance is judged according to how closely it approaches some established standard, e.g., the "ideal" care plan for a patient with esophagitis described in a case study. A standard could also be based on the previous performance of a specific group of students on the same measures, such as a previous class's performance on National Board minitests. It might also be derived from the performance of all students in a current group taking a test, e.g., an emergency-care problem-solving exercise administered to one group of physician-assistant students. Grading concepts usually associated with norm-referenced measurement (5) are appropriate in these cases, since students are expected to demonstrate different levels or degrees of proficiency in meeting developmental competence objectives.

Because of the nature and requirements of these three general factors—i.e., minimal and developmental competence objectives, their associated assessment procedures, and concomitant grading approaches—it is inappropriate for teachers to use one or another criteria system exclusively throughout a course or unit that involves both types of objectives. During the planning stage, then, teachers must consider the objectives they have established, the subject content to be addressed, and the learning activities available to students in order to determine whether a criterion- or norm-referenced approach, or a combination of both, is most applicable to specific assessment plans. The approach decided on will guide the subsequent selection and development of procedures for assessing student learning.

FORMATIVE AND SUMMATIVE ASSESSMENT OF STUDENT LEARNING

When the general criteria for evaluation have been determined, teachers can begin to select specific techniques for collecting evaluation information describing student learning.

An approach to selecting specific assessment techniques that also serves as a quality-control check on other planning activities begins with the construction of one or more tables of specifications. A table of specifications is most often described as a two-way chart depicting the relationship between learning objectives and subject content (16). While its construction is usually recommended for individual assessment devices, as will be described later, it is also useful to identifying such relationships on a course or unit basis to guide the total assessment planning process.

Tables of specifications used in the planning process are constructed by dividing a course according to preestablished units or sections, content areas, or major topics. The learning objectives for each unit are then classified by level, i.e., minimal or developmental competence, and by function, i.e., cognitive, affective, or skill. Continuing the process with the remaining units provides the same information for each, as well as a view of the course as a whole.

With a course tabled by units or other divisions, the teacher begins to decide which assessment applications are most suitable for satisfying various evaluation information needs. The teacher's decisions here are at a general level and involve both formative and summative considerations.

In deciding on any formative evaluation of student learning, a teacher considers whether the use of prerequisite tests, pretests, diagnostic tests, and/or self-assessment tests will best meet his or her evaluation requirements.

A *prerequisite test* is used at the beginning of a course to determine if students have the necessary background preparation for enrolling in and successfully completing the course. Although this type of assessment is not common in most programs consisting of interrelated required courses, it is a useful tool for teachers offering elective courses or courses open to students of varying disciplinary or academic backgrounds. The results of prerequisite testing can indicate whether a particular student is ready to enter the course, needs some additional work to meet one or more content or skill prerequisites, or is unprepared to take the course.

A *pretest* is also used at the beginning of the course to assess the nature of students' backgrounds as they relate to the objectives of the course. Unlike the prerequisite test, the pretest is administered to students who have already enrolled in a course; its purpose is dictated by the learning objectives and by the manner in which the course is to be developed and managed. If alternate learning experiences are available to students, for example, a pretest can be used in conjunction with an assessment of student characteristics to classify students by learning preference and knowledge of course content. It can also be used to assist students in selecting learning experiences; to determine if remedial or advanced work in a specific area is indicated; or to assist the teacher in selecting the teaching strategies most appropriate for these students. If an experimental teaching-learning approach is to be incorporated in the course or if new materials are to be used, a pretest can also serve to collect the first data elements called for by an experimental research design.

Diagnostic tests are used to assess specific learning weaknesses or difficulties students may be experiencing as a course progresses. This type of assessment serves a general function similar to that of the pretest, but its specific focus is on identifying problems or problem areas once a course is underway, so that corrective measures may be taken. A student in a physical-diagnosis course, for example, may be observed to have difficulty reading and interpreting X-rays. A short diagnostic test could be used in this instance to determine the nature and extent of the student's difficulty, so that some remedial work could be suggested. This test could be composed of items from previous tests or test sections dealing with X-ray interpretation. As with the use of the pretest, the inclusion of diagnostic assessments in a course assumes that provisions have also been made for properly utilizing their results.

Self-assessment tests provide students the opportunity to evaluate their own performance in a course as it is being conducted. They generally consist of sets of questions that represent a sampling of the learning objectives of a specific unit or content area. These questions are cast in a format similar to that used in subsequent summative examinations. Self-assessments serve a type of diagnostic purpose in that their results are used by students to evaluate their own progress, their own approaches to meeting learning objectives, and their own methods of learning. They differ from diagnostic tests in that any conclusions suggested by their results or any changes undertaken are up to the student alone; the teacher's responsibility is to serve as a resource and, as such, the teacher must remain in a nondirective role unless assistance is requested.

The decision to use any type of formative assessment of student learning is guided by the teacher's overall purposes in teaching, the approaches taken to the teaching-learning process, the learning objectives and learning activities forming the basis for the course, the type of students enrolled, and the resources and constraints affecting the development and management of the course. These factors combine to indicate the type of formative assessments most suitable for a course and the students taking it and to suggest the optimum frequency and timing for conducting formative assessment of student learning.

Summative assessment of student learning represents a summation or final evaluation of student performance. Such assessment can take place at the end of a formal course, teaching unit, or clinical rotation. It can also take place on more than one occasion; for example, a semester-long course divided into three units by subject content or by functional area could logically lend itself to three summative assessments, just as a course developed in two parts and taught by two teachers could lend itself to two summative assessments.

The factors contributing to decisions about formative assessments play an equally significant role in the planning and development of summative assessments. Of these factors, the learning objectives established for a course provide major direction, because the purpose of summative assessment is to elicit a final measure of the extent to which previously set criteria (i.e., learning objectives) have been met by students. Thus the minimal and developmental competence objectives of a course or unit dictate the nature and the format of the assessment, the number of assessments needed to adequately determine students' overall performance, the relationship of one assessment to another (e.g., a comprehensive cognitive-based examination and a final skills or laboratory assessment), and the time at which an assessment should best be administered. If possible, more than one summative assessment should be incorporated in any course, for almost all measurement tools a teacher develops are necessarily limited to scope and precision, and therefore no single assessment is adequate for identifying how well a student has met all the learning objectives of a course (3).

Once the teacher has decided on formative and summative assessments and has set a tentative schedule for assessing student learning, individual assessment devices can be constructed. As indicated previously, the closer this process is associated with specific planning activities, the more confident the teacher can be that valid and reliable results will be obtained from the assessment devices developed and used in the course.

TECHNIQUES FOR ASSESSING STUDENT LEARNING

A variety of types of assessment techniques are available for formative and summative evaluation of student performance in the health sciences. They differ in level of sophistication and measuring capacity, in the relative ease with which they are constructed and scored, and in the range of their applicability to different assessment situations. Several types of techniques have the potential for more accuracy and greater applicability to the educational approaches already discussed, however, and therefore need to be understood and made a part of the evaluation repertoire of health science teachers.

Multiple-Choice Examinations

The most common technique for assessing student learning has been the multiple-choice examination. It consists of items containing a "stem," usually a problem, statement, or question, and a set of alternative answers, only one of which is correct.

Other than the influence of tradition and external examining agencies, there are several reasons for the widespread use of multiple-choice as an assessment format. Multiple-choice items are able to measure different levels of outcomes; in fact, almost any understanding or ability that can be tested by other paper-and-pencil devices can also be tested by means of multiple-choice items (4). They are useful in testing situations where solutions to problems are not clearly true or false without qualification, but vary in degree of appropriateness (6). Further, they can be less ambiguously phrased than other types and are therefore less susceptible to chance errors resulting from student guessing (4). Another advantage is that multiple-choice items are objectively scored, by hand or by machine; thus, any potential teacher bias is effectively removed and the test results can be subjected to a wide range of statistical and analytic methods of assessment. Finally, if teachers follow established principles of item writing (see especially Gronlund and Ebel in the Unit 4 bibliography), they can be reasonably certain they will assess what they had planned.

Despite the advantages, the multiple-choice format is oftentimes inappropriate for specific assessment purposes or is misused as an assessment technique. Either of these conditions can occur, in part, because multiple-choice items are limited to verbal-level outcomes (6). Because students' responses are already structured, i.e., limited to a selection from given alternatives, this testing format can assess whether or not a student knows or understands action appropriate to a hypothetical problem situation, but not how the student would perform in an actual situation when required to seek out pertinent information before choosing from alternatives. Further, the multiple-choice test is necessarily limited in the degree to which problem solving can be engaged in or demonstrated by students, given its structure and the usual time constraints facing students in answering questions.

Multiple-choice can also be an inappropriate assessment technique when teachers fail or are unable to match test items to their purposes for testing, i.e., their specific learning objectives. It is frequently the case that a variety of levels or types of objectives are represented by different items in the same test. However, since the items are then analyzed together, yielding only one score for each student, the test necessarily neglects differences inherent in the objectives represented in the test.

Teachers can obtain valid results with multiple-choice tests if they use them only in appropriate assessment situations (which assumes a willingness to develop the necessary skills for constructing other assessment devices for other situations), are mindful of the limitations inherent in the format, and do not attribute to them assessment abilities they do not possess.

Teachers may also be more successful with this format if they establish performance standards for each test before it is given. This approach enhances not only the test development process, but the validity of the results of specific tests as well.

Any approach to setting performance levels has as its first step the development of a table of specifications. By following a table in the test construction process, teachers ensure that the relationships existing between objectives and content in their courses are reflected in their tests.

A table of specifications for a multiple-choice test covering one unit of an introductory primary nursing care course is depicted in Fig. 12.1. The figure shows the relationships between learning objectives and content areas by indicating the relative percentage of time students should have spent working on each objective. By applying the percentage time estimates to the number of items comprising the test, the teacher determines the number of multiple-choice items that should be written to represent adequately that objective on the test. In this

Age groups

Objectives	Infant	Toddler	Preschooler	School age	Adolescent	
List the number of required servings in each food group.	–	4	4	4	4	16
Define the most common nutritional deficiencies of the age group.	4	6	4	4	5	23
Describe the common feeding problems experienced in the age group.	6	6	6	6	6	30
Discuss the anticipatory guidance that should be given to parents with children in the age group.	3	5	4	2	2	16
Relate the common feeding problem of the age group to the child's developmental task.	3	3	3	3	3	15
						100

Fig. 12.1
Relationships between learning objectives and content
areas of a unit on childhood nutrition.

instance, if the test is to consist of a total of 50 items, two items should be written for the objective, "Define the most common nutritional deficiencies of the age group," as it relates to subject content dealing with the preschooler, since students were expected to spend about 4 percent of their unit time on this. The remaining questions are delegated in the same fashion.

Performance levels are established when the planning table is completed and before a test is administered to students by following any one of three basic approaches. If multiple-choice tests covering these objectives and content areas have been given in the past to similar groups of students, the teacher wishing to adopt the performance-level concept could begin doing so at the same time items from previous tests are chosen for use in the new test. This approach requires that the items from previous tests have already been analyzed, so that measures of item difficulty and discrimination (7) are available for each item. Thus, using standard measurement conventions, the teacher would select items with difficulty levels of at least 0.7 (i.e., 70 percent of students answered the item correctly in the past) to represent minimal competence objectives. The passing standard, or mastery level, of the test would then be set somewhere between 70 percent and 100 percent, depending on the teacher's purposes or the students' expertise (2, 10), or at the percentage representing the average difficulty level of the minimal competence test items. Students attaining the preestablished level would then be described as having "passed" the test or "demonstrated mastery" on it, while those who did not meet the level would have "failed" the test and would be identified as needing remedial work. In either case, student performance is judged according to standards representing learning objectives and previous performance of similar groups of students working on the same objectives.

If developmental competence objectives are also to be represented by items on the test, the teacher would select previous items with difficulty levels ranging from 0.4 to 0.6, the range of maximum discrimination between students' responses (3). Student performance on these items would then be scored separately from multiple-choice items and would be used to designate levels of individual achievement beyond the passing level—e.g., A, B, C; or "good, superior." Preestablished performance levels using average item difficulty as the mean of the distribution could be used to obtain these designations, as could standard curving procedures (6).

Another approach to establishing performance levels entails designating difficulty levels for each item as new test items are written (15). Difficulty levels here refer to the teacher's and colleagues' judgment of the relative correctness of each option of a test item. A designation scheme such as the following might therefore be appropriate for the five options written for a particular item:

Option	Designation
A	A response that should be rejected by a minimally competent student.
B	A plausible response.

C   A fail response—totally unacceptable.

D   A response that should be rejected by a minimally competent student.

E   Correct response.

In this example, options A, C, and D should be rejected by a student who has attained the minimally competent level of performance in a course or unit; this rejection then leaves options B and E from which to choose the correct answer. An item with two remaining plausible options would then be rated as a 0.5 difficulty-level item, for a 50 percent probability exists that a minimally competent student will obtain the correct answer by chance. Other items might have more or fewer plausible options, with concomitant difficulty levels:

Number of plausible options available to the minimally competent student	Difficulty-level rating of question	Correct response ratio
1	1.00	1.00
2	.50	.75
3	.33	.67
4	.25	.63
5	.20	.60

The correct response ratio for each item is used to determine the passing or mastery level of the total test. This is accomplished by adding together the ratios and dividing by the number of items on the test.

A similar approach to establishing performance levels is based on the number of fail, or totally incorrect, options for each item in the total test (11). When a test item is written, each of its options is rated as "correct," "incorrect," or "fail." As in the previous approach, an item may have any number of incorrect and/or fail options. When all items have been constructed, the "fail" options in each are checked off and the reciprocal of the number of remaining options is written next to the item. Thus, if option C were checked in the previous example, ¼ would be written next to that item. The sum (M) of all reciprocals is the "guess score" of a student who has just enough knowledge to reject all the "fail" options in the test.

The passing score (P) is then found by using the following formula*:

$$P = M + \sqrt{N}$$

where N is the number of items comprising the test.

Any of these approaches to constructing multiple-choice tests and establishing performance levels necessarily requires a substantial time commitment by

---

*From Leo Nedelsky, *Science Teaching and Testing* (New York: Harcourt Brace Jovanovich, Inc., 1965), p. 183. Reprinted by permission.

teachers, as well as assistance from colleagues whenever possible. The results far outweigh the effort expended, however, for these approaches can help ensure that individual items relate to learning objectives and subject content and that the total test validly assesses student learning by judging it according to preestablished criteria reflecting the learning objectives of a course or unit.

Simulation Exercises

Simulation-gaming activities can be effective teaching-learning tools, as described in Chapter 6. Simulation exercises, a variant of these activities, can also be effective for assessing developmental competence objectives that require students to demonstrate diagnostic or clinical problem-solving abilities.

The simulation exercise, or patient management problem (8), presents students with a description of a patient problem and requires them to gather data and select appropriate interventions and management techniques. Students proceed through the problem by one of several routes, which become available as the result of decisions they make. This progression is directed in much the same way as is programmed instruction and includes brief feedback or extended commentary on student decisions, along with directions for further steps to be taken.

The simulation assessment format is like the multiple-choice format in that it is structured and necessarily confined to the verbal level of performance. By providing students with several series of alternatives throughout the problem, it deviates from the actual clinical situation in that students have information they ordinarily would not know and would have to obtain from the patient or other individuals. Further, for practical considerations, this format cannot include all the real-life or situational factors that could conceivably confront students as they engage in the problem-solving process.

Despite these limitations, the simulation exercise is closer to reality-based assessment than other paper-and-pencil formats and can accommodate very effectively both minimal and developmental competence learning objectives. It is an effective format for assessing students' clinical problem-solving abilities, for it brings together factual material, a variety of data and data sources, choices of appropriate and inappropriate action, and a sequence of decision points placed in the context of an actual diagnostic-treatment situation. It is structured and standardized, so that students can compare their performance to what is recognized by their teachers as acceptable professional performance. By the same token, student performance is quantifiable, so that its analysis and interpretation is greatly simplified.

Simulation exercises are applied best to clinically oriented learning objectives, for they assess a student's abilities to bring together and utilize in problem solving material from diverse resources. They reveal how well a student is able to gather and interpret data, discriminate between appropriate and inappropriate action, choose from alternatives and make decisions, and reevaluate the situation at several stages in the process (8).

Teachers can prepare simulation exercises using only written materials; or, they can incorporate computers, videotapes, and/or slide-tapes. The basic approaches to designing and constructing simulation exercises are somewhat similar to those already discussed for simulation-gaming activities and programmed instruction; specific approaches and procedures are detailed in resources commonly available to health science teachers (see especially McGuire et al. in the Unit 4 bibliography). Reading such resources is requisite to developing written simulations. Practice is just as important, as is the assistance of someone knowledgeable in simulation construction techniques.

Basically, in developing an exercise, teachers first decide on the exact nature of the patient problem and the specific aspects of relevant decision making they want to assess. This is done, in part, by considering the set of minimal and/or developmental competence objectives that are to be represented in the exercise and by selecting clinical problems of which they have some firsthand knowledge. They then divide the intended exercise into sections relating to specific decisions to be made and develop facts, clinical or laboratory data, or other information needed to arrive at a correct or incorrect decision. This is a building process, much like that undertaken in any other development activity.

When the process has been completed, the nature of the facts, data, or other information given and the types of decisions required along the way together influence the scoring procedures to be used and the performance levels they suggest. A common scoring procedure is based on the following scheme (9):

Points	Definition
+2	Choices that are *important* at this stage.
+1	Choices that are *helpful*, although less critical.
0	Choices that are genuinely *optional*.
−1	Choices that are clearly *useless*, although harmless.
−2	Choices that are clearly *harmful* at this stage.

A performance standard, by which individual student performance can be judged, is obtained by computing a clinical management index (9). For each section of the exercise, the available decision options are rated according to what teachers and their colleagues agree is the optimum strategy at that stage of the problem. The optimum pathway(s) through the problem-solving exercise is given the highest cumulative numerical score, which is then treated similarly to student scores for comparison purposes.

Student scores for each section are obtained in the form of a diagnostic index (9), which represents the sum of option values chosen by a student divided by the sum of all positively weighted options in that section of the problem. This index, which can be compared to the management index already established, reflects the amount of appropriate information selected during the problem-solving process, as well as the relative usefulness of that information.

Because amount of information may sometimes have little relation to a student's treatment or management selections, provisions should be made for students to explain their rationale for various decisions, such as specifying the problem or reason for which particular diagnostic tests were chosen or classifying problems in terms of how urgently therapy is needed (1). This allows teachers to determine why students made or failed to make certain decisions, thus enabling them to diagnose more completely each individual student's strengths and weaknesses.

Essay Examinations

Essay examinations—and a modified version, the oral examination—are used to assess the manner and extent of student achievement of learning objectives. They require that students engage in various forms of problem solving; formulate a response that represents the results of their problem solving; and express themselves by presenting their response in written or verbal form.

Essay questions can elicit responses ranging from two to three sentences to multipage answers, depending on the nature of the objectives they represent. They are accordingly classified as either restricted-response questions or extended-response questions (6).

A restricted-response question limits the content and/or the form of a student's response. Students are directed to formulate their answers according to specific questions, as in the following example:

Describe the use of the histoplasmin skin test and serologic tests in the laboratory diagnosis of histoplasmosis.

Here, student responses are restricted in content to two types of procedures. Their ability to answer necessarily entails an understanding of the disease in question, of the two laboratory procedures, and of how the procedures can be applied to disease identification.

An extended-response question allows students to take their own approach to thinking, problem solving, and formulating and expressing a response. Teachers use this form when interested in assessing students' abilities to engage in complex behaviors, such as organizing, evaluating, and integrating, and to combine the behaviors in their problem solving. The following extended-response question is intended to assess students' understanding of cutaneous disease and its treatment:

Provide a differential diagnosis, plan an appropriate work-up, and discuss short- and long-range management of a nineteen-year-old female patient with acne.

Both the restricted-response and extended-response essay question can play an important role in a teacher's plans for assessing student learning. No other paper-and-pencil format calls on students to demonstrate the same type of abilities or elicits the same type of responses. This role can be a successful one, despite some of the limitations inherent in the essay format. These include a limit on the number of objectives and amount of subject content that can be sampled, a considerable time commitment for scoring responses and providing feedback to students, and the difficulty usually encountered in establishing and maintaining the reliability of scoring standards (6).

The effect of the first limitation can be minimized by incorporating essays as a part of a systematic assessment plan, in which other formats are utilized in concert to assess students' achievement of different types and levels of objectives. This implies that teachers develop a facility for constructing different assessment formats, understand their uses and limitations, and match them with appropriate objectives.

The effect of sampling limitations can be reduced by consulting the table of specifications constructed for the unit or section of the course and identifying the objectives and content areas best suited for assessment by essays. Restricted-response essay questions are appropriate for many minimal competence objectives; their format allows many questions to be posed in one examination. The extended-response essay is most appropriate for developmental competence objectives; its use should thus be judiciously planned to complement other assessment devices.

The time limitation is not easily reconcilable, but can be minimized somewhat if teachers and their colleagues cooperate in scoring each other's examinations. This cooperative effort should be directed by preestablished scoring criteria and performance standards, which in themselves help to overcome the limitations associated with reliability.

Scoring criteria are established before administration of restricted-response essays by first developing an outline of an ideal answer to each question, and then assigning points or credit values to the major parts of the ideal answer. These points then comprise the key for later scoring and, together, form the standard by which each student's total examination performance is judged. Because they correlate with the agreed-on major parts of ideal answers, they also help focus the scorer's attention directly on the substance of a response rather than extraneous bluffing or rambling. By first agreeing with colleagues on the rationale and the value of these points, the teacher can be reasonably certain that scoring and judging procedures will be objective and reliable.

Because extended-response questions are intended to give students considerable latitude in formulating a response, performance criteria should also address the quality of students' responses, i.e., relevance, organization, analysis, and clarity (13). While qualitative criteria necessarily entail more subjective judgment on the part of the scorer, guidelines for their application can be agreed on before scoring takes place (e.g., "Students' organization must be based on the problem-oriented medical record").

The oral examination is a variation of the essay format. Instead of requiring students to present their responses in an acceptable written format, the oral examination involves face-to-face confrontation between a student and teacher in a testing situation. It requires the ability to "think on one's feet" and to verbalize responses formulated soon after a question is asked. Oral examinations have traditionally been used in medical education for student case presentation. Having outlined the examination in rough form before the testing occurs, teachers adopt an impromptu approach during the session itself, developing the questioning according to the student's responses.

The oral examination can also be used in other circumstances in the teaching-learning process, such as at the end of a tutorial, as part of contingency contracting, or as a make-up or alternative assessment tool. If this format is used in these circumstances, however, teachers should take the same approach to developing questions as they do with a restricted-response essay question—in other words, carefully develop questions, structure the students' responses in content or form, determine ideal answers to those questions, and finalize scoring procedures before the examination is given. The examination itself is best administered by following procedures similar to those of the structured interview, wherein the interviewer leads the respondent through a series of questions, allowing no opportunity for deviation from the protocol of the interview (14).

Projects

Projects give students the opportunity to engage in complex behaviors over a specified period of time. Some product, such as a paper or laboratory preparation, is the end result of their efforts and provides the basis for assessing their performance.

The assignment of a project to be completed during a specific time is most appropriate for assessing developmental competence objectives that require a synthesis of diverse abilities, a substantial time commitment, and a product or end result that cannot be assessed easily or adequately by other formats. A project may involve a concentrated time commitment, such as a student-produced casting in a preclinical restorative-dentistry class. It may also involve an extended time commitment, such as developing and implementing a plan of care for a specific client as part of a pediatric experience in an occupational-therapy curriculum. Identifying, gathering, and coding available community resources related to VD detection as part of a preventive-medicine course is another example of a project requiring an extended time commitment.

Regardless of the setting or the anticipated product, the use of projects requires that some form of performance criteria be established before the project is assigned and that students are fully aware of the criteria before they begin the project. The criteria chosen will necessarily relate directly to the developmental competence objectives being assessed and should permit students to demonstrate creativity and originality in completing their products. Thus, the type of criteria associated with the extended-response essay question would be most appropriate for projects, for this type of criteria includes global, substantive characteristics as well as qualitative characteristics.

Performance Observation

The observation and recording of student performance in naturalistic settings comprises a major evaluation responsibility of many health science teachers. Whether conducted in a clinical or laboratory setting, this form of assessment ideally focuses on complex cognitive, skill, and attitudinal behaviors and samples a variety of student performances over time. It can serve a formative evaluation function in those instances where teaching stems from the diagnostic uses made of its results, as when students begin clinical applications of scaling and curettage. It can also serve as a summative evaluation in those instances where teachers certify student competency, such as at the completion of the clinical experience in periodontics.

Like the other assessment formats discussed, performance observation should be conducted systematically. Several general principles of assessment, if observed, can contribute to the systematic use of observational assessment. Individual teachers can modify and apply these as best fits the requirements of their own setting.

Teachers prepare for assessment by establishing performance criteria for the work setting in which students will be functioning. These criteria are usually stated as competencies students are expected to demonstrate in the setting. They reflect behaviors or components of procedures, processes, functions, or demeanors that the teachers and their colleagues have agreed are critical. It is important that all professionals potentially concerned with the setting agree on these criteria, since different individuals have slightly different ways of conducting themselves in their professional roles. A nursing-fundamentals course, for example, could be team taught by five nurses, one with a background in pediatrics, one in rehabilitation, two in medical-surgical nursing, and one in psychiatric nursing. As leaders of small groups of nursing students, then, their orientations conceivably could be based on five different approaches to procedures and management routines.

Teachers functioning in the same work setting must therefore cooperate in delineating performance criteria appropriate for the setting. Criteria can be established in light of research results in the area, common clinical experiences, and professional approaches recommended in the textbooks or the professional literature of the area. Teachers should try to be as comprehensive as possible when developing their initial listing of criteria; this initial listing is then examined for redundancies, potential ease of observation in the actual setting, and relevance to both learning objectives and the functions and requirements of the setting. The revised listing forms the basis for an evaluation try-out period, with all team members participating in using the criteria to assess student performance. A final set of performance criteria can be determined after necessary modifications suggested by the try-out experience are completed.

An integral part of the criteria development and try-out process is the selection of a method for rating student performance. Generally, a checklist approach is used to indicate whether a student has or has not met the criteria or to indicate the degree to which the student has met them. The rating method can then be based on a two-category scale, such as "satisfactory/unsatisfactory," or on a multicategory scale, such as "superior/satisfactory/correctable/uncorrectable." The choice of scale depends on the way teachers compromise between assuring agreement among raters (best achieved with a two-category system) and eliciting detailed information about student performance (best achieved with a multicategory system, i.e., four to five categories) (12).

A separate category, such as "no opportunity to observe," should also be included for each performance criterion or competency to be assessed. Oftentimes circumstances limit the nature of the experiences students can engage in. For example, although facility in various forms of written communication may be included as a competency of the setting, the activities on a specific day might be limited, as a result of institutional scheduling, to other skill areas.

In determining both criteria and rating method, teachers' decision making can be aided by considering the level of the students expected to function in a setting. Beginning students need detailed feedback on their performance, especially when starting a new laboratory or clinical routine. An observational performance assessment should therefore relate to each possible step students would cover as they engage in a procedure or process, since the formative, diagnostic aspect of evaluation is most important for them. Advanced students, on the other hand, should be able to work through procedures far more easily, often as if by second nature. Performance assessment methods would then require fewer checkpoints, but perhaps increased emphasis on such factors as original problem-solving abilities.

Provisions should be made in any performance assessment for comments. In an assessment used primarily for diagnostic purposes, comments serve to note particular strengths and weaknesses of students. While the teacher's recording of comments may serve as the primary impetus for change in student performance, when it is needed, provisions for students to add their own comments to the assessment can contribute to the press for change. Such provisions not only allow for self-assessment, they also enable students to compare their own judgments of their performance with those of professionals.

REFERENCES

1. BERNER, ETA S., LEWIS A. HAMILTON, JR., AND WILLIAM R. BEST. "A New Approach to Evaluating Problem-Solving in Medical Students." *J. Medical Education* 49 (1974): 666–672.

2. CARLSON, JOHN G., AND KARL A. MINKE. "Fixed and Ascending Criteria for Unit Mastery Learning." *J. Educational Psychology* 67 (1975): 96–101.

3. CRONBACH, L. J. *Essentials of Psychological Testing*. 3d. ed. New York: Harper & Row, 1970.

4. EBEL, ROBERT L. *Measuring Educational Achievement*. Englewood Cliffs, N.J.: Prentice-Hall, 1965.

5. GLASER, ROBERT, AND ANTHONY J. NITKO. "Measurement and Learning in Instruction." In Robert L. Thorndike, ed., *Educational Measurement*. 2d ed. Washington, D.C.: American Council on Education, 1970, pp. 625–670.

6. GRONLUND, NORMAN E. *Measurement and Evaluation in Teaching*. 2d ed. New York: Macmillan, 1971.

7. HENRYSSON, STEN. "Gathering, Analyzing, and Using Data on Test Items." In Robert L. Thorndike, ed., *Educational Measurement*. 2d ed., Washington, D.C.: American Council on Education, 1970, pp. 130–159.

8. MCGUIRE, CHRISTINE H., AND DAVID BABBOTT. "Simulation Technique in the Measurement of Problem Solving Skills." *J. Educational Measurement* 4 (1967): 1–10.

9. MCGUIRE, CHRISTINE H., LAWRENCE M. SOLOMON, AND PHILLIP G. BASHOOK. *Construction and Analysis of Written Simulations*. New York: The Psychological Corporation, Harcourt, Brace, Jovanovich, 1976.

10. MILLMAN, JASON. "Passing Scores and Test Lengths for Domain-Referenced Measures." *Review of Educational Research* 43 (1973): 205–215.

11. NEDELSKY, LEO. "Absolute Grading Standards for Objective Tests." *Educational and Psychological Measurement* 14 (1954): 3–19.

12. NUNNALLY, JUM C. *Psychometric Theory*. New York: McGraw-Hill, 1968.

13. PAYNE, DAVID. *The Specification and Measurement of Learning Outcomes*. Waltham, Mass.: Blaisdell, 1968.

14. PAYNE, STANLEY L. *The Art of Asking Questions*. Princeton, N.J.: Princeton University Press, 1965.

15. STONE, HOWARD L., HARRY J. KNOPKE, AND GREGORY A. BEHLING. *The Minimal and Discriminating Competence Examination Development Program*. Madison: University of Wisconsin Center for Health Sciences, 1976.

16. TINKLEMAN, SHERMAN N. "Planning the Objective Test." In Robert L. Thorndike, ed., *Educational Measurement*. 2d ed. Washington, D.C.: American Council on Education, 1970, pp. 46–80.

13
ASSESSING THE TEACHING-LEARNING PROCESS

Evaluation of the teaching-learning process entails specifying, collecting, and analyzing information for the purpose of decision making. Evaluation of material resources, teaching-learning activities, or the teacher's contribution to the teaching-learning process can take place in a variety of forms and provide information for a variety of decision makers. Decisions to be made using the results of evaluation can be formative, i.e., resulting in revision or refinement to increase effectiveness; or summative, i.e., resulting in the adoption or rejection of whatever has been evaluated. Formative and summative evaluation may share techniques and approaches and may occur at similar times in the educational process; they differ in the types of information they provide and in the types of decisions they engender.

To assist effectively in decision making, evaluation information must be *useful* and *usable*. Information is useful when it relates directly to the purpose of the activity or materials being evaluated. A test whose items are referenced to the learning objectives accompanying a videotape on the radiographic anatomy of the head and neck will be useful in determining the effectiveness of the videotape as a learning resource. Another test whose items elicit the recall of various pieces of information contained in the tape will be less useful for making the same determination.

Evaluation information is usable when it complements the resources available to the person in a decision-making role. A teacher responsible for two sections of a basic science course, whose department cannot provide computer time or the services of resource personnel, will be unable to collect attitudinal, descriptive, and achievement information periodically to evaluate a set of learning packages. While all these forms of information would be highly desirable for a comprehensive evaluation of the learning packages, it would be impossible for this teacher to make intelligent use of the information obtained. At the other extreme, a teacher responsible for a small group of students who has computing resources available would be remiss in collecting only descriptive evaluation information obtained from a brief checklist. While this information could be processed easily and quickly, it would be relatively unusable for rational decision making, providing a poor substitute for the variety of information that could have been obtained.

Formative and summative evaluation information must be both useful and usable to those responsible for decision making. Teachers evaluating the teaching-learning process and its parts will therefore want to plan and conduct the examination and diagnosis phases of evaluation in a manner that provides straightforward and yet comprehensive information and that complements the resources at their disposal. Decisions regarding specific evaluation approaches may sometimes be more difficult to make than those that must be made when the evaluation process is nearing completion.

Three types of evaluation information needs are associated with the teaching-learning process: those concerning material resources, those concerning teaching-learning activities, and those concerning the teacher's contribution to the teaching-learning process. Each of these information needs can be met by one or more sources of information: students, the teachers themselves, teachers' colleagues, and practitioners. In conducting either formative or summative evaluations of the teaching-learning process, the teacher must determine which sources or combination of sources will provide the most useful information, as well as which types of information will be most usable.

MATERIAL RESOURCES

Material resources are the tools the teacher develops to complement or supplement the activities of the teaching-learning process. Resources can include such things as instructional media, the elements of a course syllabus, or learning packages. Because material resources are an integral part of the teaching-learning process and contribute greatly to its overall effectiveness, teachers should, as a matter of course, obtain evaluation information describing the relative effectiveness, utility, or efficiency of the resources they use. These kinds of evaluation information can be obtained from any one or any combination of the four general sources of evaluation information, i.e., students, teachers, teacher's colleagues, and practitioners (Fig. 13.1).

Students can provide evaluation information about material resources in a variety of ways. Perhaps the most useful information they can provide, which none of the other sources can, is performance or achievement information. A series of slide-tapes used as alternatives to lectures, materials gathered together for student use on an independent-study basis, or a learning package intended to be used eventually by a variety of students: these and other resources can be

Sources	Information
Students	Performance information.
	Reactions to resources.
	Participation in experimental studies.
Teachers	Observation of student use.
	Professional opinions.
	Costs, cost benefits.
Teacher's	Professional opinions.
colleagues	Costs, cost benefits.
Practitioners	Professional opinions.

Fig. 13.1
Types of evaluation information provided for material resources.

evaluated using information describing the nature of student learning resulting from their use.

Any item or questions constituting an assessment of student learning must be referenced directly to the objectives of the resource being considered and must represent all the learning objectives rather than a sampling of them (2). If one of the objectives of a slide-tape program on streptococcal diseases calls for students to differentiate the microscopical appearance of the three main types of hemolytic reactions, test items must be directed at students' ability to differentiate alpha-, beta-, and gamma-hemolysis. Items directing students to list the cultures used to isolate and identify streptococci or classify the microorganisms found in normal and infected throats would be directed only at students' ability to recall specific information, and would thus neglect assessment of the learning objective.

The concepts of minimal competence and preestablished performance levels are integral to assessing student learning resulting from the use of material resources. The implementation of these concepts in the form of some assessment device implies that the teacher has thoughtfully conceived and carefully constructed the device. Any of the procedures described in Chapter 12 could be used to develop test items and performance levels in this manner. If a performance level of 0.75 is arrived at for a particular examination, for example, the teacher can reasonably expect the resource to be effective as a learning tool for a particular group of students if they meet or exceed that level on the examination. Additional testing of other students, with similar results obtained, would serve to confirm the resource's effectiveness, as would testing situations structured according to some experimental research design.

Students can also contribute evaluative information about some material resource during the process of its development. When a resource has reached the stage of being usable—for example, when a series of slides has been synchronized with the audiotape of a script—students can be asked to use the resource in its present form in much the same way as they would the final product. Instead of using the resource independently, each student would use it in the presence of the teacher-developer and engage in a form of oral problem solving (5). The student verbalizes the thought processes employed in working with the materials, expresses any difficulties encountered, and notes any technical deficiencies, such as ambiguities, errors, or auditory or visual distractions. By following students' verbalized thinking processes, the teacher can determine how closely the material resources match those processes, as well as discover any technical deficiencies or weaknesses in presentation that had not been previously noted.

Students can also provide evaluation information about material resources through responding to questionnaires or checklists. A questionnaire consists of a series of questions or statements intended to elicit students' opinions or reactions. Students' responses can be descriptive (e.g., short answers to open-ended questions) or quantitative (e.g., a numerical rating based on a seven-point Likert-type response scale). By responding to questionnaires, students can provide factual information—for example, responses to the statement, "Describe any changes you feel are needed in the format of this learning package." Students can also provide attitudinal information—for example, responses to a set of adjective pairs in a semantic differential scale indicating their feelings after completing an independent-study learning experience. The type of information to be collected from students is dictated by the teacher's purposes and resources.

Several general guidelines can be used for constructing questionnaires intended to meet most evaluation purposes. The first part of a questionnaire is its *set of directions.* Directions have, of course, a significant impact on the manner in which the rest of the questionnaire will be approached by those responding to it. They should clearly and concisely describe the purpose of the questionnaire, the preferred methods of responding to its questions or statements, and any additional information the respondent needs to know before proceeding—for example, the directions might identify sections where subjective comments are requested. As with many other forms of communication, what an individual wants to say in writing directions may not be what comes across to others reading them. Therefore, teachers preparing questionnaires should have them reviewed before final duplicating occurs, preferably by someone similar to those who will be responding to the final form, e.g., a student, as well as by someone who has developed expertise in questionnaire construction, e.g., a colleague.

The *layout* of the questionnaire also plays a major role in the quality of responses it elicits. The arrangement of directions, headings, questions or statements, and spaces for responses should be as simple and straightforward as possible. Teachers may be tempted to cram excessive amounts of material on a single page to save paper or to de-emphasize the length of the questionnaire. This attempt at frugality generally leads to a confusing, concentrated layout wherein every available bit of space is used. While conserving paper and limiting the length of a questionnaire are legitimate concerns, teachers should consider that open space and neat arrangement in a questionnaire are appealing to respondents, giving them a sense of freedom and creating a relaxed mental atmosphere for providing their responses.

The *scaling procedures or response patterns* used on a questionnaire should be appropriate to its purpose and to the resources available to the teacher. Generally, some form of numerical response scale is used in questionnaire construction. Tabulated numerical responses form the skeletal framework of the questionnaire's results, while any descriptive comments obtained contribute corroborating or complementary information. If the teacher must hand tabulate questionnaire responses, a "yes-no" response format is the easiest to process. If computer assistance is available or if the teacher can reserve additional time for hand tabulation, a multipoint response scale provides quantitative information amenable to a variety of analyses. Multipoint scales are usually similar in format to that of the following example:

1	2	3	4	5	6	7
Strongly agree						Strongly disagree

Respondents using this scale would be requested to choose a number from it that most closely represents their opinion or attitude toward a specific statement or question. Scales are generally anchored at each end by two opposite adjectives or statements; sometimes each numerical point on the scale is also given a descriptive label to further structure responses.

If constructed properly, the questionnaire can be an effective means for obtaining a variety of types of evaluation information. Detailed suggestions for questionnaire construction are given in several of the resources included in the Unit 4 bibliography.

The checklist can also be an effective means for obtaining descriptive evaluation information from students. A checklist consists of a listing of specific characteristics, qualities, or features of a material resource. Students are asked to indicate whether each characteristic is present or absent in the resource by placing some form of check mark in front of the characteristic listed. After viewing a newly produced videotape on the examination of the breast, for example, students could use a checklist to comment on the technical qualities of the videotape, such as color, pacing, visual displays, and narration. Teachers could use the information obtained during a tryout period as the basis for revisions of the videotape.

The questionnaire and the checklist can both provide useful and usable evaluation information. The questionnaire is generally more flexible than the checklist in that it can elicit a variety of types of information; thus, it is an appropriate instrument for use in research situations. The checklist, while limited to providing descriptive information, is easier to construct than the questionnaire and its results are more easily analyzed and interpreted. Teachers should consider the use of both types of evaluation devices when seeking students' evaluations of material resources.

Evaluation information obtained from achievement tests or questionnaires can also be collected from students participating in an experimental research study involving specific material resources. Such an evaluation is appropriate when it is necessary to generalize the learning outcomes from one group to a population of students. A department which has developed a set of learning packages for use as alternatives to lecture-discussions, and which anticipates its use by departments in other institutions, must be able to state that student learning resulting from use of the packages is equal to or greater than that resulting from participation in conventional activities. To be able to make such a statement implies that the department has randomly assigned students to one or the other teaching-learning activity and has vigorously attempted to control any extraneous factors that might have an effect on student learning.

By randomly assigning students to experimental and control groups and by attempting to control extraneous factors, teachers achieve this same effect in their teaching settings: they identify the true effects of some object or material on a sample of subjects representative of a larger population. A research design is used to ensure that true effects are not mistaken for or confused with the effects of extraneous factors. Extraneous factors cloud the true effects of a material resource and therefore cast doubt on its validity. Several factors can negatively affect the validity of a material resource (4). Some common ones that can usually be controlled in classroom research include the effects of *maturation*, or those changes that occur in students as a function of the passage of time; the effects of *history*, those changes that occur as a result of unrelated, rival events that take place during the testing period; the *reactive effects of testing*, whereby a pretest or the first use of an evaluation instrument affects the way students subsequently respond when using a resource; the effects of *instrumentation*, whereby changes or scores can vary as a result of the observers or raters themselves; and the effects of the *selection* procedures used to group students who are to use both the new and the conventional materials.

These and other factors affect the validity of material resources, either alone or in combination with one another. After deciding which factors have the potential for exerting the greatest negative effect on the material resource being evaluated, the teacher designs and conducts an experimental study to control for those factors. References included in the Unit 4 bibliography describe in detail approaches to identifying relevant extraneous factors and designing appropriate experimental studies.

Teachers themselves are valid sources of evaluation information about material resources. They are able to comment on the behaviors and performance observed of students using a resource, to respond to checklists referring to characteristics of a particular resource, and to describe the costs associated with a resource.

When developing a material resource for student use, the teacher has in mind one or more possible approaches to using the resource; several operations, mental or physical, students will perform in using it; and one or more objectives to be achieved by its use. These characteristics, operations, and expectations should be recorded during the development process, so that the teacher can use them later as checklist criteria while observing students using the resource in trial-run settings. A teacher may be interested in student reactions to the format of the resource or its mode of presentation; the time it takes students to complete their use of the resource; or the extent to which they require the teacher's assistance in completing the activities associated with the resource. While the information to be obtained varies, the procedures for collecting evaluation information are similar to those employed in evaluating students in the clinical or laboratory settings.

Some schools, departments, or groups of teachers may develop a set of standard criteria to use in evaluating material resources during the process of their development. Desired characteristics of a particular type of resource are agreed on in advance of any development activities; the characteristics then provide general guidelines for both resource development and evaluation. One basic-science department, for example, may want to begin the development of media materials for students to use on an independent-study basis. Another department may want to purchase media materials for use with large groups of students attending a departmental lecture series. Before any involvement in media production or purchasing, members of both departments should agree on the general characteristics media resources should possess, e.g., their format, degree of flexibility, mode of presentation, or the extent of personal involvement they require of a teacher. These desired characteristics will be somewhat different for both departments, because of the differences in their purposes for using media. Thus, the characteristics both departments agree on become the criteria of a checklist rating that can be used to evaluate media resources on the basis of both groups' needs.

Teachers must be able to document the costs incurred in producing or purchasing material resources for use in the teaching-learning process. Information concerning such costs are needed by teachers, their colleagues, and other decision makers, such as budget committees, who are involved in evaluating the production or purchase of resources. Few teachers have the luxury of drawing upon unlimited funds when developing material resources; most have limited budgets to work with and must therefore be quite selective and careful in their approaches to materials development.

A careful approach to materials development includes documenting either the purchase price or the direct development costs of a resource, which might include author's expenses; materials, design, and reproduction expenses; or any fees or charges associated with an external producer-director or a subject-content expert advising on specific facets of the resource (8). Indirect costs—for example, those related to maintenance of materials or equipment or the time needed to familiarize colleagues, staff, and students with use of the new resource—should also be considered when documenting the total anticipated costs of a particular material resource. While some indirect costs are likely to be less precise in their documentation than direct costs, since they are often based on estimation or projection, they hold both short- and long-range implications for the developers, funders, and users of the resource and therefore should contribute to its total costs description.

A total of the direct costs involved in producing or purchasing a particular resource is usually more meaningful to teachers and other decision makers if considered in terms of the projected use of the resource in the teaching-learning process. One method of examination entails computing the financial outlay per student per time period required to produce the resource (8). This cost figure is obtained by dividing the total direct costs of the resource by the average time students take to use it, and then dividing this quotient by the number of students using the resource during a particular time period, e.g., unit, semester, rotation.

The cost of producing or purchasing a material resource is one important type of information used in evaluating it. Another type of cost-related evaluation information, associated with the outcomes or effects of the material resource, is cost-benefit or cost-effectiveness information. Cost-benefit information describes the relative effectiveness or efficiency of some material resource compared to another. It is usually obtained through use of some form of experimental research design that examines student achievement, student attitudes, the costs of using a resource, or the amount of time students spend in using a resource.

Cost-benefit information is interpreted in terms of the expectations or philosophy of a teacher or department. A new material resource, such as a videotape, generally costs more than the conventional resource it is intended to replace, such as a textbook. New resources are purchased or developed, however, with the reasoned expectation that their effects will at least equal or exceed the effects of the conventional resource. Thus, while a videotape may cost more initially than printed materials, it can be used repeatedly by more students, in more locations, and perhaps with better results than a textbook or other printed materials covering the same subject content and directed at the same objectives.

Cost-benefit information can deal with a variety of factors, depending on the type of resource, the way it is to be used, and the purposes it is to fulfill. A teacher interested in the cost-benefit of a learning package may want to identify any improvement in the quality of learning that results from use of the package. In other words, although its direct costs may be the same as those of conventional resources, its effectiveness may be greater. Improvement in the quality or effectiveness of learning may be indicated by fewer dropouts or recorded incompletes, improved attitudes, or better student performance. It may also be evidenced by students' achieving the same learning objectives in a lesser amount of time or by students with varied backgrounds and abilities meeting pre-established performance levels, a phenomenon that would be unusual when using other resources. Cost-benefit information may also describe the efficiency of a resource; for example, as compared to another resource, it may accommodate more students, require less time or financial commitments, or permit more flexibility in the teaching-learning process.

A *teacher's colleagues* can contribute to the evaluation of material resources in much the same way as the teacher: by responding to checklists or question-naires referring to characteristics of the resource in question and by describing the costs or cost benefit of the resource.

Teachers should come to rely on the advice, reactions, and opinions of their colleagues when developing material resources for a course or unit of study. These can be obtained through use of checklists or questionnaires comprised of specific characteristics of the resource. The optimum mechanism for obtaining colleague evaluation is a formal system of colleague review established by individual departments, divisions, or schools. The system should include the evaluation not only of material resources, but also of teaching-learning activities and individual teacher's contributions to the teaching-learning process. The evaluation of material resources in a formal colleague review system should be based on criteria developed by teachers of a department or division working together. Solicitation of colleague evaluation would then be standard procedure and participation in such evaluation activities would be an accepted educational responsibility of all teachers in the department, division, or school.

In situations where formal review systems are not operating, informal colleague evaluation can be obtained by asking one or more fellow teachers to respond to checklists constructed for specific resources. Fellow teachers with subject-content or production expertise can contribute useful and usable evaluation information. Thus, these individuals should first be identified, their interest in cooperative evaluation activities established, and procedures for obtaining their evaluation agreed on.

A teacher's colleagues might also be asked to verify information regarding costs and the cost benefit of resources. While all teachers are not expected to possess the technical expertise required for costing, cost analysis, and determining cost benefits, they can provide independent verification of the costs associated with material resources and can comment on the experimental design used to assess the relative effectiveness of a new resource compared to a conventional strategy. Colleagues should be included in the financial evaluation of material resources from the beginning stages of resource development.

Health care practitioners can also contribute to the evaluation of material resources. They can offer their advice, reactions, and opinions about specific resources, particularly as a resource relates to the learning objectives the teacher has established and to actual practice situation requirements.

A checklist or questionnaire would be the most efficient and effective means of obtaining evaluation information from practitioners. For example, a slide-tape program on nutrition developed for use by medical, dental, and nursing students might be evaluated by an area epidemiologist, a public-health nurse, and a representative of the local or regional dental association. Each of these practitioners could be asked to respond to a checklist containing slide-tape criteria deemed desirable by the teacher-producer's department. They could also be asked to comment on related aspects of the slide-tape presentation, such as specific content or mode of presentation. Such practitioner evaluation might reveal community resources the teacher-producer had overlooked and failed to include in the program. Or, it might indicate approaches or practices described in the program that deviate somewhat from those used in the community by practitioners. This kind of evaluation information could thus be used to guide subsequent development activities.

TEACHING-LEARNING ACTIVITIES

Teaching-learning activities form the substance of the teaching-learning process. They include the strategies for teaching and for learning that teachers and students employ to achieve the learning objectives of a course or unit of study. Teaching-learning activities vary from course to course and department to department, for they are based on the specific purposes, resources, and constraints each teacher identifies when planning to teach. One course, for example, may consist almost entirely of lecture-demonstration as a teaching-learning activity, while another may consist of a variety of alternate activities directed at different types of students. Regardless of the specific types of activities teachers incorporate in their course or unit, the four general sources of evaluation information should each be considered when evaluation of teaching-learning activities is planned (Fig. 13.2).

Sources	Information
Students	Reactions to specific activities. Participation in experimental studies.
Teachers	Observation.
Teacher's colleagues	Observation.
Practitioners	Observation.

Fig. 13.2
Types of evaluation information provided
for teaching-learning activities.

Students are intimately involved in the teaching-learning process; they therefore have one of the best perspectives on the activities comprising it and can be expected to provide useful and usable evaluation information. The most common and most efficient means of obtaining information from students are the checklist or questionnaire. Depending on the teacher's resources, either type of device can be used to collect valid and reliable information. Further, various kinds of checklists or questionnaires can elicit specific types of worthwhile information. Questions or statements can be directive, e.g., requesting short responses to open-ended statements; or inferential, e.g., using attitudinal measures to characterize students' positions on a topic. Either of these approaches can assist the teacher in obtaining valid evaluation information from students (7).

Well-constructed evaluation instruments are essential to obtaining valid evaluation information from students. Indicating to students that evaluation results will indeed be used, and demonstrating this use during the course of the teaching-learning process, is the second major requirement. If students are convinced of the teacher's interest in their evaluation of teaching-learning activities, they will provide valid information directly relevant to the course (3), regardless of their individual predilections, attitudes, or performance levels (6).

Students participating in controlled experimental situations or in research studies also can provide valid and reliable information about specific teaching-learning activities. Such information is essential for a teacher's summative decision making about alternate activities. Because of the potential effects of the various extraneous factors on the validity of an activity introduced into the teaching-learning process, teachers should as a matter of course set up controlled situations to determine the effectiveness of new strategies or activities. The measurement of the performance and attitudes of groups of students using learning packages and groups attending lecture-discussions, for example, can help to validate the effectiveness of learning packages used by one or more different types of students. Such information is useful for subsequent planning, development, and management activities; for colleagues considering using such a strategy; and for individuals with budgetary discretion who may ultimately decide whether the development of learning packages should be encouraged and continued.

Teachers can provide evaluation information regarding teaching-learning activities by observing students and responding to checklists similar to those developed to evaluate material resources. A checklist used to evaluate some teaching-learning activity would consist of criteria reflecting the activity's desired characteristics. For example, when developing a preclinical laboratory, a teacher usually has in mind several purposes such a laboratory will fulfill, as well as specific procedures or processes students are expected to follow. These purposes, procedures, or processes become the teacher's criteria for evaluating the effectiveness of the laboratory as a preclinical experience for students. By responding to a checklist while observing students in the laboratory, the teacher records for later use some written reactions to the activity. Teachers find that written reactions are more helpful than nonwritten observations, for the latter can easily be forgotten or confused when the time comes to make any necessary revisions in the activity.

Teacher's colleagues can also provide evaluation information in the teaching-learning area by responding to structured checklists and offering any additional comments they feel are pertinent or potentially helpful. Colleagues experienced in working with different types of students or in using different types of teaching-learning activities may provide very useful evaluation information for a teacher using new or unfamiliar strategies. A colleague invited to observe students' case-study presentations and discussions, for example, may respond to a checklist detailing the teacher's expectations for the student-led sessions. The colleague may also be able to contribute additional suggestions about working with specific types of students or about alternate activities the teacher may or may not have considered in the planning and development stages of teaching.

Health care practitioners are underutilized when it comes to providing evaluation information about teaching-learning activities. Practitioners can be excellent sources of information and are often more than willing, if their time schedules permit, to become involved in the teaching-learning process in one way or another.

By observing specific teaching-learning activities and then responding to a checklist or engaging in a postactivity discussion with the teacher, a practitioner can provide information and unique insights not available elsewhere. An invitation might be extended to a hospital administrator, a staff physician, or a director of nursing from a local hospital to attend a simulation game on the institutional politics of hospitals. The practitioner may be able to make observations that can substantially improve the quality of the exercise, e.g., suggestions for altered game plays or additional role responsibilities. Such suggestions may not have been obtainable from other sources.

TEACHER CONTRIBUTIONS

Each teacher's personal disposition, demeanor, and expertise form the basis for planning, developing, managing, and evaluating the teaching-learning process. This infusion of "self" dictates the nature of the process, the way it is conducted, and the general results it can achieve. Several aspects of the teacher's self can be evaluated as they contribute to the teaching-learning process, among them attitudes toward the relationship with students, selection of teaching and learning strategies, and construction and use of devices to assess student learning. Each of the four sources of evaluation information can provide input on the teacher's contributions to the teaching-learning process (Fig. 13.3).

Students are able to distinguish between the teacher's personal contributions and other facets of a course or unit (10) and are quite capable of evaluating the impact of those contributions on their own learning. Again, if they have reason to

Sources	Information
Students	Reactions to contributions to individual learning.
Teachers	Self-analysis.
Teacher's colleagues	Observation. Inference.
Practitioners	Observation. Inference.

Fig. 13.3
Types of evaluation information provided for teacher's contributions
to the teaching-learning process.

believe the results of their evaluations will have some impact, students will take time to carefully evaluate a teacher's contributions. Further, the evaluation information they give, regardless of the type of questionnaire or checklist used, will bear no relationship to their individual predilections or performance levels (7). Teachers can therefore be confident that evaluation information obtained from students is valid and reliable, and thus useful for revising or refining the contributions they make to the teaching-learning process. If interpreted within the context of a specific course or unit, these evaluations may also be useful for other decision makers, such as department chairmen or promotions committees.

Teachers themselves can provide useful evaluation information about their own contributions through some form of self-assessment. Self-analysis of teaching usually takes place with the cooperation of experienced colleagues or educational consultants. It can occur during the teacher's regularly scheduled teaching activities or as part of a microteaching experience, wherein a specific teaching-learning activity is conducted with a small group of students in a short period of time. Self-analysis of teaching can serve to enhance a teacher's awareness and acceptance of personal strengths and weaknesses, develop a teacher's appreciation for alternative teaching styles or methods, and help the teacher to recognize the need for improvement where indicated and to develop better relationships with students (1).

Approaches to the self-analysis of teaching are usually based on the pattern developed for microteaching. In microteaching, a teacher works with a colleague or consultant in a laboratory-type environment; conducts a single teaching-learning activity, which is usually videotaped, with a small group of students in an allotted period of time, e.g., fifteen minutes; has the activity critiqued by the colleague or consultant; and then conducts the activity once again with another group of students. This cyclical teach-critique-reteach pattern not only serves to identify strengths and weaknesses, it demonstrates improvement in the teacher's performance, which over an extended period of time can be significant (9).

A variety of approaches to self-analysis is available to teachers. In an optimum situation, opportunities for self-analysis should be made available by a department, division, or school for interested teachers. In a less-than-optimum situation, teachers might seek out experienced colleagues willing to serve as observer-consultants. Resources have been included in the Unit 4 bibliography which detail approaches to microteaching and self-analysis. Teachers should be able to find in them a specific approach to meet their current needs and fit the resources at their disposal.

Colleagues can evaluate a teacher's contributions to the teaching-learning process through observation and through inferences drawn from the performance of the teacher's students. In both cases, colleagues can provide useful and usable evaluation information, whether the procedures for providing such information are formalized in a colleague review system or are conducted on an informal basis by several teachers.

Colleagues can assist a teacher's self-analysis through microteaching or through observing a teacher in actual situations and responding to a questionnaire or checklist. Colleagues with expertise in developing various assessment devices, in using different teaching strategies, or in managing different types of students can provide evaluation information to complement or supplement that obtained from other sources. Colleague evaluation freely requested and freely given can be invaluable, whether for new teachers beginning their teaching duties, for experienced teachers trying new strategies, or for experienced teachers who want to improve their handling of educational responsibilities.

A teacher's contribution to the teaching-learning process can also be assessed by colleagues through the inferences they draw from the performance of the teacher's students. Students' grasp of fundamentals can be noted by a colleague responsible for teaching a subsequent course or unit; similarly, students' skills in clinical problem solving developed through use of simulation exercises can be readily identified by cooperating clinical teachers. These and other behaviors or performance characteristics of students can be observed by colleagues and their observations, whether on a formal or informal basis, can assist the teacher in subsequent planning, development, management, and evaluation activities.

Health care practitioners can also evaluate a teacher's contributions to the teaching-learning process through observing the teacher in an actual teaching-learning situation or through inferences drawn from student performance. Most teachers are reluctant to solicit peer evaluation, much less evaluation from practitioners. This reluctance is usually the result of an institution's approach to evaluation. If evaluation is seen as a positive, rather than negative, activity, however, both colleague and practitioner evaluation can be freely requested and freely given.

Practitioner evaluation of a teacher's contributions to the teaching-learning process, particularly as a role model for students, can be given through observation of the teacher in actual teaching-learning situations. By becoming familiar with the specific learning objectives of the session or activity and by following a checklist of desired characteristics, practitioners can provide useful and usable evaluation information based on their professional perspectives. Such information will complement and supplement that obtained from other sources.

Practitioners can also evaluate a teacher's contributions through inferences drawn from observing the teacher's students. Practitioners in preceptor roles, in clinical supervisory roles, or in consultative roles may have the opportunity to work to some degree with a teacher's students. Feedback on student performance offered on a formal or informal basis will be of value to teachers in their subsequent teaching activities.

REFERENCES

1. ADAMS, WILLIAM R. et al. "Research in Self-Education for Clinical Teachers." *Journal of Medical Education* 49 (1974): 1166–1173.
2. ANDERSON, R. C. "How to Construct Achievement Tests to Assess Comprehension." *Review of Educational Research* 42 (1972): 145–170.
3. BAUSELL, R. BARKER, STANLEY SCHWARTZ, AND ANAL PUROHIT. "An Examination of the Conditions under which Various Student Rating Parameters Replicate across Time." *Journal of Educational Measurement* 12 (1975): 273–280.
4. CAMPBELL, DONALD T., AND JULIAN C. STANLEY. *Experimental and Quasi-Experimental Designs for Research.* Chicago: Rand McNally, 1963.
5. CUNNINGHAM, DONALD J. "Evaluation of Replicable Forms of Instruction: A Classification of Information Needs in Formative and Summative Evaluation." *AV Communication Review* 21 (1973): 351–367.
6. FELDMAN, KENNETH A. "Grades and College Students' Evaluations of Their Courses and Teachers." *Reseach in Higher Education* 4 (1976): 60–111.
7. GREENWOOD, GORDON E. et al. "A Study of the Validity of Four Types of Student Ratings of College Teaching Assessed on a Criterion of Student Achievement Gains." *Research in Higher Education* 5 (1976): 171–178.
8. LAWSON, TOM E. *Formative Instructional Product Evaluation*, Englewood Cliffs, N.J.: Educational Technology Publications, 1974.
9. OLIVERO, JAMES L. *Micro-Teaching: Medium for Improving Instruction.* Columbus, Ohio: Merrill, 1970.
10. ROMNEY, DAVID. "Course Effect vs. Teacher Effect on Students' Ratings of Teaching Competence." *Research in Higher Education* 5 (1976): 345–350.

14
REQUIREMENTS FOR USING THE RESULTS OF EVALUATION

Evaluation activities are conducted to obtain information useful for decision making. The manner in which a specific evaluation activity is developed and conducted has a direct effect on the way in which this information can be used.

If a systematic approach is taken to developing and conducting any evaluation activity, the results obtained almost always are valid and reliable. Valid results are those that serve the purpose for which they were intended; reliable results are those that are stable or consistent, or those that can be generalized from one group or situation to a similar one. Any teacher engaged in evaluation should focus on obtaining valid and reliable results, for such data can be used without hesitation as the basis for decision making in the prescription phase of evaluation. If a simulation exercise assesses the clinical problem-solving skills it was intended to assess, and does so consistently, the results it provides can be used for judging student performance. Similarly, if student evaluations represent stable assessments of teaching-learning activities, the results of their evaluations can be used in judging the effectiveness of the teaching-learning process.

Validity and reliability are two of the most important factors determining the ultimate usability of evaluation results. Without them, a teacher cannot be certain of the quality of the information available, and therefore has a questionable basis for making decisions. Validity and reliability should therefore be routinely established for any evaluation activity.

VALIDITY

Validity is a function of the purposes of an evaluation activity. Test results may be valid when used to describe graduate pharmacy students' mastery of specific learning objectives; the same test, however, would more than likely produce invalid results if used to predict the performance of first-year students entering the pharmacy curriculum. Similarly, the results of an evaluation of media materials may be valid for formative decision making, but less valid for summative decisions. The validity of evaluation results must thus be assessed and interpreted in the context of the purpose of the evaluation activity.

Teachers may encounter three general kinds of validity when conducting evaluation activities: content, criterion-related, and construct validity (6). Content validity refers to the extent to which evaluation results are relevant to the objectives, content, or attributes being evaluated. Content validation is usually accomplished through some judgmental process in which the evaluator and colleagues assess the relevance of the measuring device to whatever is being measured.

Criterion-related validity refers to the relationship between evaluation results and one or more external factors known or believed to represent the characteristic, behavior, or attribute being assessed. An entrance examination, such as the ACT, SAT, or MCAT, is judged according to the extent to which the test is useful for predicting students' later academic performance. Academic performance, usually measured by grade-point average, is the criterion against which students' test results are judged. In these cases, criterion-related validity is essential, for admissions committees rely on the results of such tests to be predictors of students' later performance in their educational programs. In a classroom situation, a performance test intended to predict first-year family practice residents' community diagnostic skills would have criterion-related validity if the scores of practicing physicians who had taken the same test were available for comparison. The practicing physicians' test results would represent the standard or criterion against which the residents' results would be judged. Correlation or regression procedures are usually chosen to determine criterion-related validity.

Construct validity refers to the psychological qualities assessed by an evaluation device; it indicates the degree to which some theoretical or explanatory construct explains the evaluation results obtained. A teacher in a traditional curriculum may be interested in assessing students' motivational levels at various times during their independent work with learning packages. Using the process theory of motivation as a guide, the teacher develops a questionnaire to be administered to students at designated intervals of a unit. The extent to which the results of the questionnaire correlate with the various factors or constructs of the process theory represents the questionnaire's degree of construct validity. Correlation or factor analysis procedures are most often used in the construct validation of an evaluation instrument.

Each type of validity plays and important part in a comprehensive system of evaluation. As teachers develop in their roles as teachers and as their evaluation activities become more comprehensive in scope and character, they must at the same time develop expertise in assessing and identifying each type of validity as it relates to the various purposes of their evaluation program. However, teachers should be concerned first with establishing the content validity of their evaluation activities. Content validation is appropriate for any evaluation activity teachers conduct, from achievement tests to assessing specific teaching-learning activities. It is also basic to the other types of validity. By establishing content validity on a routine basis, teachers can be reasonably certain that the evaluation information they obtain will be useful for decision making.

Content validation of a test, attitude inventory, or course evaluation is a judgmental process; it entails determining the extent to which an evaluation device assesses the objectives, attributes, or subject content intended to be measured. The validation process begins with a careful delineation of the *purposes* of the evaluation activity, the *objectives, attributes, or content* intended to be measured, and the *criteria* to be used in analyzing the responses obtained by the evaluation device. The delineation of these factors provides the criteria the teacher and one or more colleagues use in judging the relevance of the items, questions, or statements to whatever is being measured. The degree of agreement achieved among judges indicates the extent to which the evaluation device is valid for its intended purpose.

Validity is based on an analysis not only of the format of an evaluation device, but also on an analysis of student responses to it. A validation procedure that can be used with student responses to tests referenced to minimal competence objectives involves examining the degree to which test scores discriminate between a group of students that has mastered the objectives and a group that has not (2).

It can be assumed that a group of students engaged in teaching-learning activities directed toward a specific set of objectives contains a high concentration of students who develop mastery of the objectives. Similarly, it can be assumed that another group not involved in teaching-learning activities directed at the objectives contains a high concentration of students who do not develop mastery of the objectives. The validation procedure is based on these assumptions. The pass-fail scores of two groups of students, one receiving instruction toward the objectives and the other not receiving it, are compared to provide a validity index for the test. The index is found by analyzing scores of the two groups using the following formula (2)*:

	Uninstructed group	Instructed group
Pass	B	A
Fail	C	D

$$\text{Validity index} = \frac{(A+C)}{N}$$

$$\text{where } N = A + B + C + D$$

*From Kevin G. Crehan, "Item Analysis for Teacher-Made Mastery Tests," *Journal of Educational Measurement* 2 (1974): 256. Copyright 1974, National Council on Measurement in Education, Inc., East Lansing, Michigan. Reprinted by special permission.

If a test has been developed carefully to reflect the objectives of a course or unit and its content has been validated by one or more judges, this additional validation procedure corroborates that the information obtained from the test is indeed useful for identifying students who have mastered specific objectives.

An additional procedure that can contribute to the validation of multiple-choice test items referenced to either minimal or developmental competence objectives involves examining the difficulty and discriminating indices of each item. *Item difficulty* represents the percentage of students who answer the item correctly; it ranges from 0.0 (all answered incorrectly) to 1.0 (all answered correctly). *Item discrimination* represents the ratio of students scoring highest on the entire test who answer a specific item correctly to the students scoring lowest on the entire test who answer the item correctly. It ranges from -1.0 (all of the lowest-scoring students answered it correctly, all of the highest-scoring students answered incorrectly) to $+1.0$ (all of the highest-scoring students answered correctly, all of the lowest scoring students answered incorrectly) (3).

A minimal competence item would be expected to be answered correctly by most, if not all, students if they have mastered the objective it represents. The percentage of students answering the item correctly should therefore equal or exceed the minimal performance level established for the test. If the performance level of a test is set at 0.8, for example, students should be expected to meet or exceed this level if they have mastered specific learning objectives. Similarly, their performance on each item should be expected to be at least close to this overall performance level if each item is functioning as intended. An item whose difficulty index is much below this level, e.g., 0.6, is not functioning as expected and is therefore invalid for the purposes of the test.

There should be little or no discrimination among students' scores on a minimal competence examination, as all students would be expected to at least meet the minimum performance level. Each item should therefore have a very low positive discrimination index, or none at all, if it is functioning as expected. An item with a high positive or a negative discrimination index may not make a valid contribution to the entire test, particularly if its difficulty level is below the pre-established performance level of the test.

A developmental competence item is written to discriminate between students of varying abilities and is intended to determine the extent to which students have approached achievement of developmental competence objectives. Maximum discrimination between students is achieved when an item has a difficulty level in the 0.4 to 0.6 range. A difficulty index much below this range, e.g., 0.21, indicates the item is very difficult and may not be measuring in the manner it was expected to measure. A difficulty level much above this range, e.g., 0.79, indicates the item is too easy and not able to discriminate students' performance.

A developmental competence item should have a high, positive discrimination index, for if it is functioning as intended, it should be answered correctly by students who score highest on the whole examination and incorrectly by students who score lowest. A small, positive discrimination index or a negative one indicates the item is inadequate; it is misleading or misrepresenting itself to students and thus is not discriminating in the manner intended.

The use of item-analysis statistics provides teachers with an additional validity check of multiple-choice tests used to assess student performance. If item-difficulty and item-discrimination indices for a specific item indicate the item has not performed as anticipated for the group of students taking the test, the item is invalid for assessing the performance of that group. It should be omitted from further consideration and should not be included in student scores; otherwise, the validity of the entire test may be adversely affected.

RELIABILITY

Reliability represents the stability, consistency, or generalizability of evaluation results. Like validity, reliability is directly related to the purpose of an evaluation activity. Unlike validity, it is entirely a statistical property of the results of evaluation. The procedures for establishing reliability for a particular evaluation activity must therefore be chosen in accordance with the purpose of the activity.

Procedures for determining reliability can be as precise and as sophisticated. as resources permit. If computer time and consultants are available, for example, teachers can routinely submit evaluation results to high-powered, sophisticated analysis procedures. If resources are limited, procedures are available for teachers to compute reliability themselves. The reliability obtained may not be as precise as that obtained by computer, but it will give a usable estimate of the actual reliability of evaluation results.

When using standard analysis techniques to determine the reliability of an assessment of student performance, reliability is usually based on the amount of variation found in student scores. In general terms, the more variation in scores, and the more scores approximate a normal (bell-shaped) distribution, the higher the reliability will be. These techniques are appropriate for tests assessing developmental competence objectives where variation is expected; they are not as appropriate for tests assessing minimal competence objectives, where variation is not expected. If most or all students demonstrate mastery of objectives, there will be little variation among them in their test scores and, hence, a reliability value obtained by standard procedures will give an inaccurate picture of the test's reliability.

A procedure that can be used for estimating the reliability of teacher-made tests assessing students' achievement of minimal competence objectives involves comparing students' performance on two parallel tests. The procedure is based on the assumption that if a test is consistent in its measurement of specific objectives, students should perform equally well (or poorly) on both forms of the test.

A reliability estimate is obtained by comparing the proportion of consistent individual mastery decisions for a group of students on the two tests. The students who equal or exceed the preestablished performance level of both tests are compared to those who fail to meet that level on both, using the following formula (2)*:

Form B

		Fail	Pass
Form A	Pass	B	A
	Fail	C	D

$$\text{Reliability} = \frac{(A + C)}{N}$$

$$\text{where } N = A + B + C + D$$

This formula can be used easily by teachers in analyzing the tests they construct to assess student achievement of minimal competence objectives. While not as powerful or sophisticated as other procedures for determining reliability, it is appropriate for tests where little variation or discrimination among student scores is expected. It requires little time and no computer resources to calculate and it provides a reasonable estimate of the reliability of a minimal competence test.

Most teachers have available to them some form of testing or test-analysis service through which their developmental competence examinations can be analyzed and scored. The majority of these service agencies employ the Kuder-Richardson method for determining reliability (7); this is a powerful technique, based on the amount of variation present in student scores. If teachers have the opportunity to participate in the development of a new or altered testing service, however, either within their own school or department or within their institution, they should consider using the Hoyt method of determining reliability (4). The Hoyt method is algebraically equivalent to and just as powerful as the other major methods. Because this method employs the analysis of variance statistical techniques in arriving at a reliability coefficient, it can provide more information to the teacher about characteristics of a test than can the other methods. Using analysis of variance permits the identification of the amount of variation that exists among the items of the test, as well as the amount of variation that exists among student responses to the test. Such information, when combined with traditional item-analysis information, can be used by teachers for both formative and summative decision making about student performance in a course or unit.

Procedures for determining the reliability of objective-based assessments of student learning provide a quantitative measure or estimate of reliability. Similar procedures and quantitative results are not available for subjective-based assessments, e.g., extended-response essay questions or project reports. The reliability

---

*From Kevin G. Crehan, "Item Analysis for Teacher-Made Mastery Tests," *Journal of Educational Measurement* 2 (1974): 256. Copyright 1974, National Council on Measurement in Education Inc. Reprinted by permission.

of such assessment forms cannot be computed directly, but can be enhanced by the manner in which the assessments are analyzed. A four-step approach to the analysis of subjective assessments of student learning serves to enhance reliability by reducing the potential for error in rating such assessments (1).

The first step entails the use of a sufficiently fine scale for rating student responses. A rating scale is used first as the basis for establishing minimal performance levels before the assessment is conducted, and later for scoring student responses. A general rule of thumb is that a rating scale having from seven to fifteen points or units provides useful and reliable information.

The second step of this approach requires that clear reference points be developed to anchor the rating scale. To be consistent in scoring answers to essay questions, for example, the teacher needs to have a clear idea of the meaning of each point of the rating scale. Thus, each should be defined. The more precise the definition, the more reliable the teacher's subsequent ratings of student responses are likely to be.

The third step consists of rating responses to subjective assessments question by question, rather than student by student. By rating all responses to the same question at once, the potential for introducing systematic error into the rating process is reduced. If all of one student's answers on an essay examination were rated at once, for example, the impression made on the teacher by an answer to one question may influence the rating of answers to later questions.

Finally, the teacher can reduce the potential for error due to personal bias and increase the reliability of scoring procedures by having one or more colleagues assist in the rating of student responses to subjective assessments. Teachers who cooperate in the scoring of each other's assessments in general obtain more reliable ratings than a teacher working alone. Such cooperation necessitates the careful delineation of the purposes, criteria, and scoring procedures of the assessment.

The reliability of most evaluation activities, e.g., questionnaires, attitude inventories, or checklists, concerned with the teaching-learning process or its parts can be established easily by teachers. If computer facilities are available, coefficient alpha (5) is perhaps the most versatile and most precise method available. If reliability must be computed without the use of a computer, the coefficient of reproducibility (8) can provide the best estimate of the reliability of evaluation results.

Coefficient alpha provides a measure of the internal consistency of an evaluation device. It is algebraically equivalent to the Kuder-Richardson and Hoyt methods of determining reliability and is based on both the average correlation among the items of the evaluation device and the number of items comprising it. Because it provides an assessment of internal consistency, coefficient alpha can be thought of as the expected correlation between an actual evaluation device and a hypothetical parallel form, one that is not constructed. The reliability of the results of a course evaluation or attitude inventory can be determined using coefficient alpha, for example; the resultant reliability estimate represents the upper limit of the reliability of the results. Computing split-half reliability for the course evaluation or attitude inventory—i.e., dividing an instrument in half and correlating both halves as if they were parallel forms of a particular evaluation device—provides an even lower reliability estimate.

Coefficient alpha is sensitive to the sampling of the items constituting the evaluation device and to the various sources of error that are present in specific evaluation situations. Because of this sensitivity and because of its power to provide an upper bound of the reliability of evaluation results, coefficient alpha should be the preferred method for teachers developing a comprehensive evaluation system.

If computer resources are not available, the coefficient of reproducibility can easily be calculated by teachers to determine the reliability of the results they obtain from using questionnaires, attitude inventories, or checklists.

An estimate of the reliability of evaluation results is obtained by following a three-step procedure. First, the teacher and one or more "judges," e.g., colleagues or graduate assistants, categorize the responses to each item of the evaluation device according to whether or not the responses strictly agree with each other. Intermediate categories of partial agreement or partial disagreement are not considered. The answer or point on a response scale that respondents chose most often becomes the criterion for judging agreement or disagreement. Thus, the following distribution of responses to an item using this scale:

	Strongly agree					Strongly disagree	
Response scale:	1	2	3	4	5	6	7
Number of responses:	5	25	6	2	0	0	0

would result in 25 responses categorized as "agree" responses, because they represent the scale point most often chosen, and 13 as "disagree" responses, because they differ from that criterion of agreement.

The categorized responses for each item are then used to compute the coefficient of reproducibility, using the following formula (8)*:

$$\text{Coefficient of reproducibility} = 1 - \left[\frac{\text{Number of disagree responses}}{\text{Number of items} \times \text{Number of respondents}} \right]$$

---

*Reprinted by permission from Samuel A. Stouffer et al., *Measurement and Prediction* (Gloucester, Mass.: Peter Smith, 1973).

The resultant coefficient represents the extent to which the obtained responses approximate the hypothetical perfect distribution of the attributes, attitudes, or opinions in question. Coefficients of reproducibility near or above 0.90 have been shown to be efficient approximations to perfect distributions, i.e., the evaluation results they represent can be considered to be reliable.

When the coefficient of reproducibility has been computed, the lower bounds of the reliability of individual items can be estimated by using the following formula (8)*:

$$p \geq \frac{m}{m-1} \left(r - \frac{1}{m} \right)$$

where p is the lower bound of the item's reliability, m is the number of categories of responses to the item, and r is the coefficient of reproducibility. It has been shown that item reliability is at least equal to this obtained lower bound, but is almost always higher (8).

REFERENCES

1. COFFMAN, WILLIAM E. "On the Reliability of Ratings of Essay Examinations." In William A. Mehrens, ed. *Readings in Measurement and Evaluation in Education and Psychology*. New York: Holt, Rinehart and Winston, 1976, pp. 93–103.

2. CREHAN, KEVIN D. "Item Analysis for Teacher-Made Mastery Tests." *Journal of Educational Measurement* 11 (1974): 255–262.

3. HENRYSSON, STEN. "Gathering, Analyzing, and Using Data on Test Items." In Robert L. Thorndike, ed. *Educational Measurement*. 2d ed. Washington, D.C.: American Council on Education, 1970, pp. 130–159.

4. HOYT, CYRIL. "Test Reliability Estimates by Analysis of Variance." *Psychometrika* 6 (1941): 153–160.

5. NUNNALLY, JUM C. *Psychometric Theory*. New York: McGraw-Hill, 1968.

6. *Standards for Educational and Psychological Tests and Manuals*. Washington, D.C.: American Psychological Association, 1966.

7. STANLEY, JULIAN C. "Reliability." In Robert L. Thorndike, ed. *Educational Measurement*. 2d ed. Washington, D.C.: American Council on Education, 1971, pp. 356–442.

8. STOUFFER, SAMUEL A. et al. *Measurement and Prediction*. Gloucester, Mass.: Peter Smith, 1973.

*Reprinted by permission from Samuel A. Stouffer et al., *Measurement and Prediction* (Gloucester, Mass.: Peter Smith, 1973).

UNIT 4
BIBLIOGRAPHY

BABBIE, EARL R. *Survey Research Methods*. Belmont, Ca.: Wadsworth 1973.

A good resource on the design, use, and analysis of survey research methods. Principles of survey research are appropriate and applicable to evaluation activities, particularly to those concerned with the teaching-learning process. Chapters on instrument design, questionnaires, interviews, and data processing are especially helpful.

CAMPBELL, DONALD T., and JULIAN C. STANLEY. *Experimental and Quasi-Experimental Designs for Research*. Chicago: Rand McNally, 1963.

A basic resource on experimental designs appropriate for educational research, particularly research conducted in classroom situations where control of all extraneous variables is not always possible. Recommended resource for any teacher engaged in the development, management, and evaluation of instructional methods or materials.

CRONBACH, LEE J. *Essentials of Psychological Testing*. 3d ed. New York: Harper & Row, 1970.

A basic reference on the principles and procedures of testing; directed primarily at standardized, norm-referenced testing and measurement issues.

EBEL, ROBERT L. *Measuring Educational Achievement*. Englewood Cliffs, N.J.: Prentice-Hall, 1965.

A standard reference dealing with most aspects of the educational measurement process. Chapters on planning a test and on constructing and using essay, true-false, and multiple-choice items are still highly appropriate and can be quite useful for health science teachers.

GRAY, CHARLES E. "The Teaching Model and Evaluation of Teaching Performance." *Journal of Higher Education* 40 (1969): 636–642.

Describes model of teaching and suggests evaluation criteria that might be used in assessing the relevancy of teaching performance. Criteria represent observable behaviors that can be identified by one who is an experienced teacher and qualified in the subject being taught. Can be useful as a general guide for student, peer, and self-evaluation.

GRONLUND, NORMAN E. *Constructing Achievement Tests.* Englewood Cliffs, N.J.: Prentice-Hall, 1968.

A straightforward, concise reference covering the preparation and administration of achievement tests. Useful guidelines for constructing mimimal competence items and essay questions.

GRONLUND, NORMAN E. *Measurement and Evaluation in Teaching.* 2d ed. New York: Macmillan, 1971.

Probably the most thorough and yet readable book on educational measurement available to teachers. Although directed at primary- and secondary-level teachers, health science teachers will have no difficulty using it and applying its principles and procedures to their own setting.

Journal of Educational Measurement (quarterly). Published by the National Council of Measurement in Education, East Lansing, Michigan. Library of Congress No. AP J83 E259.

Major refereed education journal containing original measurement research and reports of measurement in an educational context. Includes reviews of educational and psychological tests and new work on evaluation and measurement. Many of the technical papers require measurement and evaluation background, although practice-oriented papers are included. Style of the journal makes papers readable for the nonspecialist interested in the most recent work on measurement and evaluation.

Journal of Educational Psychology (bimonthly). Published by the American Psychological Association, Inc., Washington, D.C. Library of Congress No. AP J83 E26.

Major refereed education journal containing original papers concerned with the gamut of psychological issues relevant to education. Papers generally cover all areas and interests of education; can therefore be used as a continuing resource for most of the issues discussed in this book. Usually contains papers dealing with some aspect of measurement and evaluation.

KERLINGER, FRED A. *Foundations of Behavioral Research.* 2d ed. New York: Holt, Rinehart and Winston, 1973.

A basic, comprehensive resource covering most aspects of research principles, methods, and procedures used in the behavioral sciences. The sections on measurement and methods of observation and data collection should be particularly useful for teachers developing a systematic evaluation program.

LAWSON, TOM E. *Formative Instructional Product Evaluation.* Englewood Cliffs, N.J.: Educational Technology Publications, 1974.

Presents a variety of instruments and strategies which can be used as described or adopted to fit specific formative evaluation requirements. Straightforward and readable.

McGUIRE, CHRISTINE H., LAWRENCE M. SOLOMON, and PHILLIP G. BASHOOK. *Construction and Analysis of Written Simulations.* New York: The Psychological Corporation, Harcourt, Brace, Jovanovich, 1976.

One of the basic resources dealing with simulation exercises. Recommended for any teacher interested in developing an understanding of and using simulation exercises to evaluate student performances.

NUNNALLY, JUM C. *Psychometric Theory.* New York: McGraw-Hill, 1967.

A comprehensive resource on measurement theory. Some discussions are highly technical; those concerning validity, reliability, test construction, and the measurement of abilities, traits, and behaviors are generally practice oriented and quite readable.

OLIVERO, JAMES L., *Micro-Teaching: Medium for Improving Instruction,* Columbus, Ohio: Merrill, 1970.

A concise reference describing the principles and procedures of microteaching. Useful for teachers interested in developing a system of self-analysis of their teaching.

OPPENHEIM, A. H. *Questionnaire Design and Attitude Measurement.* New York: Basic Books, 1966.

A useful reference covering the development, use, and analysis of questionnaires and other evaluation devices.

PAYNE, DAVID A. *The Specification and Measurement of Learning Outcomes.* Waltham, Mass.: Blaisdell, 1968.

Pulls together research and theory on educational measurement. Contains good annotated bibliographies on each of the topics covered.

STOUFFER, S. A. et al. *Measurement and Prediction.* Gloucester, Mass.: Peter Smith, 1973.

An extensive treatment of the measurement of attitudes. A detailed discussion of reliability and the uses of the coefficient of reproducibility.

STUFFLEBEAM, DANIEL E. et al. *Educational Evaluation and Decision Making.* Itasca, Ill.: Peacock, 1971.

Report of a study which examined extant models of evaluation and generated an evaluation model intended to help practitioners improve their educational efforts. Ties evaluation to several levels and categories of decisions. Provides a useful framework for understanding the role of evaluation in the educational process.

THORNDIKE, ROBERT L., ed. *Educational Measurement.* 2d ed. Washington, D.C.: American Council on Education, 1971.

A collection of essays on a variety of issues and topics concerning educational evaluation and measurement. Combines theoretical and practical approaches to measurement. The papers it contains are generally included among the authoritative references of the area.

VAN WART, ARTHUR D. "A Problem-Solving Oral Examination for Family Medicine." *Journal of Medical Education* 49 (1974): 673–680.

Describes principles and procedures involved in the preparation and administration of a structured oral examination intended to measure problem solving. Presents a good model for oral examinations that can be adapted for use in most health science education programs.

UNIT 5
PERSONAL
MANAGEMENT

The personal role of teaching—that is, teachers as teachers—is often neglected when the teaching process is examined. The previous units have dealt with the four-stage framework of planning, developing, managing, and evaluating teaching and learning, areas that typically are covered in in-service or faculty development activities. This unit focuses on the teacher as a person and on the relationships developed with students, teacher peers, and self.

Teaching is a growth process, in which teachers are continually seeking new insights about themselves and others. By carefully observing how a teacher relates to others, it is possible to gain a better understanding of the teacher as a person. By the same token, self-analysis by the teacher allows the teacher to be more effective in relating to peers and students.

Some teachers react to discussions of student-teacher and teacher-peer relationships as "labeling," "manipulative," or "reducing the spontaneity of the relationship." Human behavior is often predictable. Knowledge of the dynamics of human behavior when applied to the student-teacher or teacher-peer relationship can only enhance the depth of understanding in the relationship. Labeling and manipulative behavior occurs only when teachers abuse the power, rights, and privileges their role confers. Managing relationships effectively does not destroy spontaneity. Quite the contrary, it maximizes the potential of any relationship.

Understanding behavior and being able to predict behavior enables teachers to manage relationships more effectively, for they know where and how best to invest their personal energies. Teachers cannot be all things to all people. Thus, it is very important for teachers to understand who they are and how they can most productively relate to students and teacher peers. Such self-knowledge can help them to experience more fully the joy of teaching.

The goal of this unit is to sensitize teachers to the important interpersonal aspects of teaching and to encourage continued growth in this area. Chapter 15 discusses teacher-student relationships, focusing on types of difficult relationships teachers are likely to encounter. Teacher-peer relationships are described in Chapter 16. These relationships may include working with peers, under peers, or with teaching assistants. A framework for managing relationships is discussed and some strategies are suggested. Chapter 17 discusses the teacher as a person and presents a format for ongoing self-evaluation.

15
TEACHER-STUDENT RELATIONSHIPS

Through the transactions of the teaching-learning process, teachers can develop different types of relationships with a group of students. The types of relationships developed depend on the teacher's personal educational philosophy. It is relatively easy to assume the role of director and tell students what they should learn, when they should learn it, and how they should learn it. This role is natural for many teachers, for it emphasizes the teacher's position as content expert and the students' position as recipient of the teacher's knowledge. It is less easy to assume the role of facilitator—that is, to develop a variety of learning experiences and then share control of learning with students. In this role, the teacher sometimes encourages students to plan their own learning activities and to make mistakes and, at other times, sets limits on students to help them conform to activities prescribed especially for them.

While teachers generally accept the fact that they are professional role models for students, they often do not realize the impact their teaching role has on students as they transact with them. The teaching role is an integral part of the total professional role of the teacher; students associate teacher-student relationships with professional-client relationships. Both the directive and facilitative teaching-learning relationships, as well as those combining elements of the two, have immediate and long-term effects on students.

MANAGING RELATIONSHIPS

Because of the nature of health science education programs, students with behavioral problems are not common. Competition and rigorous entrance requirements often effectively screen out students who could present teachers with problem behaviors. Most students are willing and eager to learn and, while they might prefer one or another type of relationship with teachers, they can participate successfully in the teacher-student relationship established for a course or unit. Still, despite the screening effect of the admissions process, many teachers at one time or another do find themselves in the position of having to manage difficult relationships with students, relationsips that deviate from those normally found in the teaching-learning process.

The unmotivated student, the immature student, the older student, the dishonest student, and the student with emotional problems all present special challenges. Before attempting to manage relationships with these types of students, the teacher must first determine why particular behaviors are being expressed by particular students. In general, student behaviors fall into two categories: behaviors related to the course and the teacher's management of it; and behaviors related to personality and developmental issues of the student. The successful management of relationships with students depends on the teacher's ability to initially assess the dynamics of the teaching-learning situation and the students' behavior in it.

The Unmotivated Student

The unmotivated student is often slow in handing in assignments and may appear apathetic in achieving learning objectives. This behavior might be related to the way in which the course is managed. The student may be reacting to a lack of structure or to activities and materials that communicate course expectations poorly. Or, the course may be structured so that different kinds of behavior are rewarded and the student cannot decide which behavior is most desired.

Developmental or personality factors could also account for this behavior. There are a number of possibilities. An unmotivated student might simply be one who is afraid to make a mistake, for any one of a variety of reasons. The process of separating from parents might have caused the student to experience some anxiety due to the departure from the comfortable home environment and the inability to get along without parental direction. Or, the student might harbor a need to be perfect, in order to fulfill the expectations of family or friends. Perhaps the course is so overwhelming to the student that intellectual immobilization occurs.

Another developmental factor that should be considered when assessing the unmotivated student is the possibility of an unrecognized learning disability. It is often thought, incorrectly, that adults know if they have a learning problem. However, such a problem may go undetected until a group of factors come together and create a learning situation that causes the student to experience extreme difficulty. Incongruent achievement represents such a difficulty and indicates that a student should be further tested for the existence of a learning problem. An example of incongruent achievement is the student who appears to know the content well, but fails an examination; or the student who fails an examination one day, but receives an A the next day on a similar form of the test.

Before planning how to intervene with the unmotivated student, the teacher needs to become familiar with some of the approaches to motivation in adults. One current approach, the process theory of motivation (1), can be a useful framework for considering motivation issues. It identifies four areas that contribute to the degree of motivation in an individual. The first concerns students' perceptions of the *likelihood that if they try they will succeed*. Students who perceive that they cannot succeed are not motivated to try. Despite a strong interest in becoming a health care professional, for example, a student who is deficient in reading skills might soon experience problems of motivation when faced with an increasing amount of written course material. Similarly, a group of students in a newly approved physician's-assistant program may have motivational difficulties if they are scheduled in basic science courses conducted by a medical school. In this area, the assessment of student characteristics, course prerequisites, and the sequencing of courses are very important factors to be considered.

The second area concerns students' perceptions of the *definition of success in the course*. Do students clearly understand the course expectations, objectives, desired skills or behaviors, and evaluation methods? Motivation is decreased when students do not understand what is expected of them. In this area, the delineation of objectives, learning activities, and evaluation methods and standards is very important.

Students need to understand clearly the *connection between level of performance and the teacher's evaluation of that performance*. Motivation is highest when students see that fulfilling specific objectives leads to personal accomplishment and satisfactory evaluation by the teacher. It is important, therefore, to link success in specific learning activities with success in the course or unit.

Finally, students must *value the content of the course and its outcomes*. Students who value the content, skills, and behaviors comprising a course will be more motivated than those who do not share that valuation. If the course is perceived as not helpful, irrelevant, or redundant, students are less likely to put their full effort into it.

Two premises have to be accepted in following this approach to motivation. The first premise is that students do those things they think will lead to satisfaction and avoid those things they think will create dissatisfaction. Thus, the student's perception is critical when teachers deal with a lack of motivation. If students think that being pleasant and coming to class with a minimal amount of preparation will produce satisfactory results, they will not be motivated to do more than that. A student for whom C is a satisfactory grade and D an unsatisfactory grade will not be motivated to do B work, but will be highly motivated to perform above D level.

The second premise is that to some students rewards are very important. If students feel they are doing what is required of the course but are not being rewarded, they will stop. By the same token, if students are rewarded when they achieve specific course objectives, they will be motivated to continue.

In managing the unmotivated student, the teacher should first be sure that the link between performance and reward is clear. Some teachers reward students for attending class instead of achieving specific learning objectives. Motivation is decreased if students perceive there is no link between performance and the rewards (feedback) they are receiving from the teacher. Rewards should also be given at the time the behavior takes place. Some students perform quite well continually, but may not receive feedback, a reward, or a positive clinical evaluation until the middle or the end of a course or unit. The unmotivated student should be given immediate feedback, but *only* for desirable behavior. Motivation quickly declines if every behavior is rewarded. Lastly, if the student is unmotivated, the teacher needs to be sure the course has a formal system of achieving rewards. Teachers often assume the only rewards needed in the course are grades. For some students this is true. But for others, verbal praise, given privately or in front of peers, may also be a reward.

Too frequently teachers assume that all students want to be challenged. They believe that, by challenging a student, they can increase that student's motivation. Challenging increases motivation only in students who have a high need to achieve. Thus, if a student does not have a high need to achieve, the teacher and the course should not be encouraging or challenging the student to an unnatural level of achievement.

Developmental and personality factors also have to be considered when assessing motivation in students. The teacher should have access to and use resources in which students can be professionally evaluated for learning disabilities and problems. There should also be remedial activities and resources for students who are identified as needing them. The student should be actively involved in discovering and dealing with the learning problems. With progress in this area, motivation should increase.

Depression can interfere with the energy a student has available to devote to course work, and the behavior that results may appear to be apathetic and unmotivated. Depression is a major health problem of adults, with suicide one of the leading causes of death among young adults. What becomes most difficult for the teacher is determining whether the cause of the apathy or lack of motivation is a significant depression in the student; frequently, this is extremely difficult to establish. If there is evidence to support the suspected presence of depression, the teacher must promptly refer the student to available professional resources. Often these resources exist within the school, but students are reluctant to pursue them themselves because they fear a loss of confidentiality.

The Immature Student

Immature students often have difficulty in concentrating, making decisions, and becoming involved in the teaching-learning process established for a course or unit. These students may be absent often and spend a great deal of energy trying to do the least amount of course work possible. They frequently lack clear-cut goals and seem to change their goals and interests often.

In assessing whether this type of behavior is a reaction to the course itself, the teacher must determine whether or not the course or its parts lack sufficient structure. Insufficient structure allows this type of student to manipulate the amount of involvement and the amount of work that is done. The course may also lack a variety of activities from which to choose. The immature student may have difficulty with small-group discussions or lectures, for example, but may enjoy a learning package or programmed instruction. The availability of alternatives enhances the possibility the immature student will be confronted with a realistic and yet challenging approach to learning.

A developmental factor that may account for immature behavior is the student's perception that areas in adult life other than education are more important at the moment. Attempts to set priorities may result in regressive or seemingly immature behavior in a student. For example, a student who is looking for a mate or one who is awaiting the birth of a first child may appear to be immature in their respective classroom behaviors. This behavior may, however, reflect a limited ability to become totally involved in an academic course at this particular time. If immature behavior is a result of pressures in other areas of the student's life, then the teacher needs to accept this behavior as the most mature behavior possible from this student at this time.

An effective way to manage immature behavior is to provide a syllabus that clearly outlines the structure, expectations, and limits of the course. Within this structure students expressing immature behavior should have an option of choosing alternate ways of meeting the learning objectives of the course. The immature student may enjoy less active, more traditional teaching-learning activities. Or, because of external pressures, this student may respond positively to a slide-tape or other activity developed as an alternative for a specific scheduled lecture.

The Older Student

A third type of student is the older student, one who might be thirty, forty, or fifty years old. A student may be pursuing a second career, such as a practical nurse entering a baccalaureate program, or returning to school for full-time or enrichment work. An "older" student might also be only twenty years old, but behave in a mature way because of significant previous learning or practical experiences. Each of these student types is self- and goal-directed. Since such direction is desirable, these students should be assisted in overcoming any obstacles blocking their goal-attainment efforts.

Mature students confront a set of obstacles somewhat different from that confronted by more traditional students. One situation that may prove troublesome for the mature student is a course that requires media or the use of some form of educational technology. Some students, particularly older, more mature students, may be unfamiliar and uncomfortable with these new learning tools. Often reading or a lecture is a more acceptable and effective way of learning for them.

Further, the course may not have pretest or preassessment tools that utilize a student's previous experience and knowledge, so valuable time may be wasted in a course that contains information already wholly or partly known to a student. It may be that the student is proficient in only a part of the course, but there is no mechanism for challenging just a part of it.

A developmental factor that can interfere with the older student's progress in a course is the requirement that all students join a group or conform to a set of expected behaviors. Wider life experience makes this conformity difficult for the older students. To manage a course where students are expected to study and meet course objectives in a rigidly prescribed way may not be possible for the older student who either questions the need for such rigidity or for whom such rigidity is a severe hardship as a result of outside pressures, such as a family or job. This student may choose not to become a part of the group.

In managing relationships with older students to maximize their learning, the teacher should first use pretest tools to assess the level of their entering skills and abilities. Contingency contracting is also helpful either in helping the student avoid redundancy within a course or in allowing the student to meet objectives in an alternate way. Group learning activities should include a variety of strategies and independent-study options should be available whenever possible.

It may be helpful at times to cluster these students, when feasible, to maximize their learning by involving them in a group. Some courses may even be specifically taught for them, although certainly these students should not be singled out nor discriminated against.

The Dishonest Student

The dishonest student presents a particularly difficult student relationship for the teacher to manage. A dishonest student may be one who reports the completion of a clinical responsibility, e.g., the administration of medications, but actually failed to complete it. A dishonest student may infrequently or never turn in assignments and be unable to answer questions on the unit, but consistently pass examinations. Dishonesty is difficult to identify and substantiate; it can be mistaken for other phenomena and it can cause awkward and even legally difficult situations. Once dishonesty has been identified and validated by the teacher, it is necessary for the teacher to determine the reasons a particular student is exhibiting dishonest behavior.

The learning management of the dishonest student depends first on whether the teacher's assessment indicates that the dishonest behavior may be in reaction to a course situation or whether it is more likely a personality factor of the specific student involved. In assessing whether this behavior is a reaction to the course situation, the teacher needs to know if the course standards are too high for the student to achieve. It may be that the student is experiencing undue pressure to achieve in a particularly difficult course. It might also be that the particular course has too many objectives or too much content for the student to successfully master.

The teacher must also determine if the dishonest behavior has occurred before. The teacher needs to ascertain if there is any pattern to the type of dishonesty being exhibited. For example, does the dishonest behavior appear at certain parts of the course, or with certain types of students? Does it seem to be related to certain types of assignments? Management for this type of behavior is then based on assessing why the undue pressure or the need to be dishonest is occurring and how the situation could be modified to relieve the pressure.

If it appears the dishonest behavior is an individual personality or developmental problem, it is very important for the teacher to have anecdotal records to support the observations and the conclusions being made. Encouraging peers at this time also to evaluate the student's behavior helps to ensure that the dishonest behavior is, indeed, a specific personality problem. Most schools have established criteria by which dishonesty, both academic and clinical, is handled. This may involve severe actions, such as removing the student from the course, the specific clinical situation, or the school. It also frequently involves an appeals process. While the teacher generally does have established guidelines to deal with this type of behavior, it is nevertheless a difficult task. However, identifying and managing this particular type of relationship is very important if teachers are to maintain professional standards.

The Student with Emotional Problems

When confronted with a student with emotional problems, although this is not common, the teacher must be able to assess human behavior accurately. It may be that the particular student behavior is one in which anxiety is overtly expressed. Anxiety, while a common phenomenon in all learners, is most significant in students with emotional problems. This student often has set unrealistically high personal standards and is constantly frustrated by an inability to function at that level. Perfection is often the goal actively sought by this type of student. The anxiety resulting from failure to achieve perfection can become so severe that it may interfere with the student's ability to function in the classroom, laboratory, or clinic.

Severe withdrawal is another behavior sometimes exhibited by a student with an emotional problem. The withdrawn student may engage in inappropriate behavior or experience problems in functioning on all levels of activity, whether intellectual, attitudinal, or skill. This type of student may not have any relationships with peers and, in fact, may be generating a great deal of anxiety in the other students in the course.

A third type of behavior of students with emotional problems stems from alcohol or drug abuse. Such students' work is erratic and may be accompanied by noticeable changes in behavior. There may be mood swings—signs of euphoria followed by signs of depression. There can also be overt physical signs: fatigue, nervousness, weight loss, and a lack of concern about personal appearance.

It is inappropriate to associate the emotional problems of students with the management of a course. Thus, the behaviors exhibited by students with emotional problems should be viewed as a reaction to their own personality factors or developmental issues.

It is very important for the student who is extremely anxious to receive a great deal of feedback and support from the teacher. When the anxiety level of this student is high, the teacher should be supportive and help the student reduce the level of anxiety, so that it does not interfere with the student's ability to function. In times of low levels of anxiety, the teacher can provide the student with feedback and help the student to begin to understand why the anxious behavior occurs and what the student can do to reduce it. An awareness on the student's part that the anxiety may be related to self-expectations and not the teacher's expectations can be quite helpful. However, if the anxiety is so high that it interferes with the student's ability to function, the student needs to be confronted with this fact and referred to an outside professional resource.

The teacher should also attempt to maintain a relationship, whenever possible, with the student who exhibits inappropriate behavior. This student may be very frightened or reject any attempt to develop a relationship. The goal of the teacher in such severe cases should be to refer the student as soon as possible to the proper source of help. The student most often encountered is the suicidal student. It may be necessary to remove this student from the course and to involve the family if treatment and/or hospitalization is needed. This is indeed a difficult situation for a teacher to handle. Teachers should identify in advance resources available to help severely disturbed students.

The student who exhibits behaviors associated with alcoholism or drug abuse needs to receive feedback about this type of behavior. The teacher should be clear in delineating the limits of acceptable behavior and should seek corroborating opinions from peers about whether or not the behavior of this student is indeed inappropriate. Students should be given feedback on how their specific behavior is affecting their progress in accomplishing academic and personal objectives. When possible, options should be suggested. However, the objectives need to be evaluated in terms of the particular behavior the student exhibits, for these students can often be manipulative in their attempts to deny their emotional problems.

REFERENCE

1. FIEDLER, FRANK E. *Leadership*. New York: General Learning Press, 1971.

16
TEACHER-PEER RELATIONSHIPS

During the course of their professional interactions, teachers develop several distinct and yet sometimes overlapping relationships. They have relationships with students and with fellow teachers. Sometimes peers may ask to audit or sit in on teachers' classes as students. Teaching assistants or faculty assistants may later be hired and then become colleagues. The role of department chairman may be a function that is elected and shared, so that a fellow teacher could easily be an administrative superior for a period of time and then a peer again. All of these situations require the teacher to be sensitive to the fact that such relationships are dynamic and that their management calls for a variety of skills.

STAGES OF RELATIONSHIPS

In managing relationships, teachers can use the framework for group life described in Chapter 10. Relationships follow the same three phases that groups follow—i.e., initiation, working, and termination. A difficulty exists in that these three stages can occur over a few weeks or several years. Therefore, at any one time a teacher may experience many relationships, each of which is in a different phase. For example, one relationship could be with a new teacher, another with a long-term colleague, and a third with a colleague who is leaving. While it is not necessary to determine the exact phase a relationship is in, it is helpful for the teacher to be aware of the common issues found in each phase, as this knowledge is useful in managing relationships.

The Initiation Phase

Experienced teachers are often unaware of the various phases of their relationships with others. For new teachers, however, the phases are more obvious. As a new teacher, one of the tasks to be accomplished in the initiation phase is to become oriented to the institution. This is facilitated in a variety of ways, from an orientation program to informal social gatherings. In some respects, the beginning of a new school year is an initiation phase for every teacher, especially if there has been a summer break. For schools that run year round, this may not be the case; other efforts will be required.

Initiating new relationships involves a great deal of anxiety for new teachers. They fear possible rejection and anxiety related to uncertainty about what the new situation will be like. New teachers often look for structure as a way to cope with this anxiety. In attempting to develop a structure within which to operate, teachers attempt to identify similar and dissimilar characteristics they share. Thus, discussions about where teachers live, went to school, or to which clinical specialty they belong are common early in the year.

The initiation phase is also a time of testing and developing trust. This testing is often done unconsciously and may take the form of the new teacher saying no to a request or refusing committee membership to see how the individuals involved react. If the behavior of the colleague teachers is predictable, then the teacher is more likely to begin to develop trust. The established teachers also test the new teacher. They might be very cautious initially, carefully revealing more and more of their own educational philosophies over a period of time until they feel fairly certain this teacher is someone to be trusted.

Many unwritten rules or standards exist within every school, such as which committee has the most prestige or if it is acceptable to leave the office early and finish work at home. Until the new teacher has caught on to these rules, many mistakes may be made during the initiation period. It can thus be a frustrating and lonely time.

New teachers often are tempted to call their previous places of employment to hear about what has happened since they left. Their secret wish is that they are sorely missed or that they can never really be replaced. They are still ambivalent about their decision to move to a new school and are likely to continue to feel this way for several more months.

The initiation phase may last a few weeks or a few months, or it may be the entire first year. This all depends on the teachers involved and how quickly they become acclimated to their new surroundings. The next phase, the working phase, begins when teachers feel they understand their roles and responsibilities. It is important that new teachers allow themselves time to become acquainted and develop these important trust relationships. In this way, teachers begin to feel they belong to the new school.

The Working Phase

The working phase of a relationship is the most difficult to describe, since the behaviors vary so greatly. However, teachers know they are in the working phase when they trust their colleagues and enjoy working with them. Teachers begin to feel productive, stimulated, and challenged. Obviously, a teacher cannot expect to trust and enjoy working with every colleague, but personal satisfaction in the teaching role is most prevalent in the working phase.

It is during this phase of a relationship that teachers are most likely to try new teaching strategies and behaviors. Teachers who attempt too much innovation, particularly before they have an opportunity to know the school and their peers, often experience significant frustration and resistance.

Change at any time is threatening to teachers, but it is particularly threatening when initiated by "strangers," i.e., teacher-colleagues not known or trusted. Even during the working phase, change can be interpreted as an indication that things were initially wrong or bad. Teachers need to change and grow continually and they need to manage their relationships with their peers so that change is interpreted as an important, necessary aspect of teaching, not an implicit judgment of how things were handled before. Change in a course or in teaching behaviors is an individual matter. So, for a teacher to implement a simulation game in a course should not imply that the previous way of covering this content was wrong. The change can more accurately be seen as a reflection of the teacher's concern about continually developing better skills in the planning, development, management, and evaluation of the teaching-learning process.

When teachers experience resistance, jealousy, or frustration as they create change, they need to assess why these feelings are present. It is difficult to analyze the causes when teachers are not yet well acquainted with their colleagues.

In the working phase, teachers know which of their teacher peers they can trust and are therefore more easily able to interpret feelings of resistance and jealousy. In fact, teachers can often predict the feelings their colleagues are likely to display. When this happens, teachers are prepared and able to handle these reactions.

The Termination Phase

Termination, or the final phase of relationships, is perhaps the most difficult phase for teachers to manage. The decision to leave is, in itself, a hard one. However, the reality is that teachers outgrow schools and a move or change in teaching positions is generally beneficial for professional growth. The fantasy of the teacher who remains in the same school for twenty-five years and who becomes the resident scholar because of this experience is exactly that—a fantasy.

The decision to stay or leave is a personal one and should be made in terms of what is best for the individual teacher, not according to what will look best on a work record. Once the decision has been made to leave, and a commitment is made to a new school, the teacher should share this information with peers. This is important, because only if the separation is expressed can peers begin to help the colleague leave.

Initially there may be some denial about leaving, expressed frequently by zealous involvement in institutional activities. Some teachers may even volunteer for extensive school projects, knowing they are leaving. Denial often is an indication of a great deal of ambivalence about leaving. However, it is to be discouraged, since it is inappropriate for a leaving teacher to participate so actively in a course or school when any decisions made will have to be implemented by another teacher.

As the separation becomes more imminent, teachers often find themselves feeling very angry. Sometimes they express this anger in comments like: "This school is sure going downhill"; "Seems like the course problems are getting worse"; or, "I'm glad I'm getting out of here before the new hospital opens!" These feelings serve to help teachers withdraw and begin to separate from the school and their peers. It would be too painful to leave a perfect school and perfect peers, so teachers often begin to find fault with both the school and their colleagues before they leave.

Just before leaving, the ambivalence that all teachers feel, no matter how glad or sad they are in leaving, can create depression. There are always good and bad feelings related to leaving a position and both types need to be expressed. It is considered much more acceptable to express negative feelings before separating, although the good feelings also need to be shared. By sharing these warm feelings with colleagues, teachers can more easily separate and go on to other teaching relationships.

TEAM TEACHING: TEACHING WITH OTHERS

Many schools utilize team teaching. It can take the form of several teachers teaching the same course because of large enrollments, but functioning relatively independently except for this fact. Another type of team teaching occurs when a master or lead teacher attempts to coordinate the efforts of the team, while every teacher still teaches all aspects of the course. The most typical type of team teaching is where a group of teachers share their expertise and each assumes major responsibility for a specific part of the course. Together they share functions of the course.

Team teaching in any form can be difficult in that it requires that many, if not all, of the decisions related to course planning, development, management, and evaluation be made by a group. Not only is this difficult, it is terribly inefficient at times. The advantage of team teaching is that experts are offering their knowledge and insights directly to students. This can be a thrilling and an engaging experience for students who are accustomed to teachers presenting material from areas outside their special areas of interest.

Some teams of teachers divide functions within the course, while others manage the course by consensus. Whatever method is most efficient and the most satisfying for the teachers involved should be used.

Even if there is not formal team teaching and even if each teacher teaches an individual course, there still is some type of organization of the faculty as a whole. This may be an organization according to the level of student being taught, e.g., freshmen, junior, or resident, or according to specialty areas, such as psychiatry, pediatrics, and obstetrics. It is through these organizations that teachers come to know their teacher peers.

THE ADMINISTRATIVE HEAD

New teachers need to establish clearly what is expected of them in terms of teaching, as well as in terms of administrative and committee duties. It is particularly important to determine the relative importance of each of these areas. For example, in one institution, teachers' primary responsibility may be teaching, while in another teachers might be expected to devote equal time to research and teaching. Some committee responsibilities are more important than others. Teachers need to determine this within the framework of their own institutions.

It is essential that the teacher have an understanding of the system within which rewards, monetary or administrative, and promotions occur. Some institutions reward teachers on a uniform basis, while others operate on a merit system. Some institutions also have a tenure system in which there may be many written and unwritten rules. Many times these rules do not directly affect the teacher during a particular year, but, in the long run, they may determine whether a teacher is allowed to continue employment within the institution.

Many teachers find that an informal written contract, in which the goals and activities of the teacher are defined for the teacher for a year, is helpful. The contract should be negotiated with the administrative person directly responsible for the teacher, such as the division or the department chairman. This person is most familiar with the particular teaching being done by the teacher and, in addition, is also the person responsible for doing the annual review of the teacher. By writing this contract together, the chairman and the teacher agree in advance on the importance of the goals. This contract then becomes the framework for the end-of-the-year evaluation. Thus, for example, at the end of the year, after putting a great deal of time and energy into course revision, a teacher can be properly rewarded and not confronted with the discouraging fact that the chairman is happy for the course revision but unhappy that committee participation was only minimal that year. Obviously teachers cannot do everything; thus, each year or semester, they need to agree in writing with their administrative supervisor on the scope and depth of their involvement.

Lastly, it is very tempting to become a member of a particular faculty, go through requisite faculty orientation, and then encapsulate oneself within a course. What this does is cut the teacher off from really understanding how the philosophy of the school is practiced. While the school's philosophy may be found in a written document, it is more accurately stated by the practices of the present group of teachers, and it is only through interaction with other teachers that this philosophy can be known. It is also important to be actively involved in teachers' meetings, since administrative decisions can significantly affect the philosophy of the school, the curriculum, and the quality of the education of the students. Thus, a good case can be made for becoming and remaining actively involved in matters of administration. It is possible for faculty members who have been associated with an institution for some time to assume an almost proprietary air with regard to the curriculum; they come to be identified with it. However, if these faculty have stopped communicating with the newer faculty or have stopped sharing the new ideas of the teachers, then they are no longer in touch with what is happening in the school. It is only through active debate among both teaching and administrative staff that a truly quality educational experience can be achieved for students.

FACULTY ASSISTANTS: TEACHING THROUGH OTHERS

A faculty assistant may be a graduate student or someone who, for whatever reason, is not prepared to assume full leadership and responsibility for a course. If a faculty or teaching assistant does not function in a teaching role, then it is possible for a teacher to relate to the assistant by assigning administrative or ancillary activities. If, however, the assistant is to perform teaching functions, such as grading papers, leading discussion groups, or leading laboratory experiences, then it is important that this person be included in the development and ongoing management of the course. That means that a weekly meeting of some kind needs to be held during which the content and course activities are discussed and management decisions are made.

Too frequently, master teachers assume that since assistants are competent in the content being taught, they are therefore competent to teach it and to make decisions related to the teaching-learning process. Even if the student or assistant has had teaching experience and coursework, it is important for the teacher periodically to discuss student problems, teaching-strategy problems (such as group discussion, laboratory, or lecture problems), and evaluation problems. These three areas—student behaviors, teaching strategies, and evaluation—are often the most difficult for teaching and faculty assistants.

When teachers allow assistants to participate in the teaching function, they still must assume the major responsibility for the teaching that students receive. Thus, if an assistant is having difficulty with a particular group of students, it is the responsibility of the teacher to intervene. The assistant should know from the beginning of the course that the teacher will provide supervision or assistance whenever necessary.

It is helpful when the course begins for the teacher and the assistant to write a contract in which the teacher clearly describes the expected behaviors of the assistant and the assistant has an opportunity to ask for certain kinds of support or opportunities to develop personal skills. This encourages both to become actively involved in the management and success of the course. If the assistant is not offered an opportunity to develop personally, then course participation becomes nothing more than another job and there is little incentive to make it a quality learning experience for the assistant or the students. If, however, the teacher agrees to help the assistant prepare and present a lecture or if the teacher agrees to evaluate periodically the assistant's group skills, then both the assistant and the students will benefit from the experience.

While weekly course-management meetings are necessary if there are teaching assistants in the course, it is also necessary to use other tools to evaluate the teaching occurring in the classroom. For example, frequent unit tests and periodic visits by the master teacher into the classroom of the assistant can be made. While some may feel this undermines the role of the assistant and may generate anxiety in the students, if handled properly, quite the opposite will be true.

The presence of inexperienced or new assistants in a course only indicates more strongly the need for peer review. However, even if there are only two teachers in a course, they should whenever possible visit each other's classrooms.

Students should be told they will have a teaching assistant, that the teacher will be periodically visiting the classroom, and that the teaching assistant is expected to visit the teacher's classroom. When students have an opportunity to see this mutual evaluation in operation, they no longer look on it as an element of the superior-subordinate relationship. It becomes clear that evaluation is necessary to make the course as beneficial as possible for every student. This greatly encourages students to become more involved in the course.

NEW SKILLS

It has become increasingly necessary for teachers to learn both research and management skills. Teachers who find themselves teaching in colleges and universities need to be sensitive to the importance of research in these institutions and to the need to be able to communicate with the other disciplines in terms of the research being conducted. Management skills are necessary for teachers who are now frequently called on to manage grants, prepare budgets, and become involved in interviewing new candidates and in establishing policy.

Another required proficiency area is that of writing and publishing. Teachers are often expected to publish in journals and to engage in other writing. It is important for teachers who decide to pursue either of these endeavors to seek help from a colleague who has already published. Such assistance can be invaluable in acquiring and developing the skills needed.

Since it is difficult to decide in advance if seeking out a colleague or taking a course in an area will provide the particular skills desired, a teacher needs to consider increasing skill proficiency by a variety of experiences. For example, a course in organizational behavior combined with a practicum experience with a hospital administrator may provide the teacher with the skills previously lacking. For another teacher, this might only be the beginning. A whole course of study or an advance degree might be necessary. In developing new skills, the teacher needs to be aware that available resources include colleagues, workshops or courses, and graduate-degree programs.

THE SCHOOL

The teachers and the administrative staff form a school which may or may not exist within a larger institution. Teachers need to be able to function within the social, economic, and political areas of these institutions. The teacher who is part of a city junior college which affiliates with various large hospitals, for example, needs to be able to function within both the milieu of the city junior college and the other large institutions, public as well as private.

When a problem arises for the teacher that relates to relationships outside of a course, the teacher should consider the possibility that the problem is a result of one of three common causes: lack of common goals and agreement; lack of understanding about the social structure of the institution; or unfair distribution of rewards (1). Certainly there are myriad other possible causes, but these three are most prevalent.

Lack of common goals and agreement can lead groups of teachers to take conflicting directions in their work. For example, one group of teachers may actively pursue introducing research content into the curriculum, while another may be attempting to increase the amount of clinical experiences for students. When the teachers come together, they realize that the plans they are proposing are incompatible, since the groups did not agree in advance on common goals. Obviously, in this situation, these two plans did not have to be mutually exclusive, but, if preliminary agreement or sharing of common goals is not pursued, this can happen.

Lack of understanding about the social structure of the institution is a common cause of problems for schools. A definite social structure exists in every student body and every faculty body, as well as in every institution. This structure is often difficult to articulate and it is constantly changing. Many professions have neglected to prepare their practitioners to relate to and be sensitive to this structure. Hence, teachers often find themselves stymied, because they have made proposals that were perhaps educationally very sound, but in conflict with the social structure of the institutions.

Unfair distribution of rewards continues to be a source of problems for many teachers. Monetary rewards can often be better distributed when faculty are actively involved in establishing peer review and criteria for promotion. However, the reality is that there are many other types of rewards, such as the teacher who gets a private office or an office with a window, or the teacher who is given support for research. Sometimes the rewards are so individual as to go unnoticed, unless care is taken to determine if this is an aspect of the problem. For example, a teacher may appear very reluctant to participate on a committee even though previous interest was expressed, simply because the teacher's name was inadvertently left off of a recent memo to the committee members.

In addition to considering the reasons for common problems, teachers should also examine institutional communication patterns (1). As teachers pursue their work goals, certain forces act to encourage them to communicate with individuals who can help them achieve their aims, while other forces act to discourage communication with those who will not assist or who may regard their efforts as unimportant. It is important for teachers to determine if a problem stems from such a communication pattern within the school. If it does, the teacher should try to identify what this pattern is, who is behind it, and why it has developed.

People direct their communication to those who make them feel more secure and gratify their needs and away from those who threaten them or make them feel anxious. Teachers need to identify what the needs of the individuals are and who may be threatening the individuals and making them anxious.

Lastly, individuals in an organization frequently communicate according to what they personally view as important—i.e., they are apt to focus most often on areas they are concerned about improving. Teachers need to be sensitive to what an individual views as self-improvement and to be supportive of that area. For example, a fellow teacher may view improvement as developing skills in teaching, while another may want to receive feedback on managing relationships within a difficult clinical area. Knowledge of this type can be very helpful to the teacher who must interact with both teachers.

The teacher, in working with several distinct groups of individuals and overlapping relationships, needs to develop skills in managing these diverse relationships. This is an important area, since the interpersonal experiences within a teaching situation can significantly affect the degree of success a teacher realizes in an institution.

REFERENCE

1. JACKSON, JAY M. "Lines of Communication." In Sandra Stone et al., eds., *Management for Nurses—A Multidisciplinary Approach*. St. Louis: C. V. Mosby, 1976, pp. 49–57.

17
TEACHER-SELF RELATIONSHIPS

Just as teachers' relationships with students and peers affect the nature of the teaching-learning process, so too does their knowledge of "self." By developing a relationship with self, teachers can come to know their strengths and weaknesses as persons and as teachers. Such knowledge helps them to formulate effective individual approaches to teaching.

In order to grow and develop, the teacher-self relationship needs to be examined continually. Assessing the teacher-self relationship involves looking at several areas and compiling data to form a personal plan for development. With first attempts to assess "self," teachers often discover they have difficulty with things that relate more to teaching than to their professional areas of expertise.

FACTORS CONTRIBUTING TO TEACHING DIFFICULTIES

The discovery of teaching difficulties should not cause the teacher to feel inadequate or hopelessly unqualified for the task. Research conducted on teacher behaviors in classroom situations has shown that most instances of poor teaching are not the result of deliberate or even conscious acts of the teacher involved. They result from a combination of factors: inadequate or inappropriate training; conditioning processes that cause bad teaching habits to become established and maintained; and lack of adequate mechanisms for giving teachers feedback to help them change their behavior (1). Thus, discovering problems is the first step toward seeking solutions and improving one's efficacy as a teacher.

Many teachers in the health sciences become teachers because they have displayed excellence in their areas of expertise. The assumption is made that a good professional is also a good teacher. In reality, these are two separate professions with two separate areas of skills. Teacher preparation may not even have been part of the professional's education. While many schools are now including in their curricula some content, often on the graduate level, related specifically to teaching and learning, and while some health care professionals are prepared in the area of teaching, most are *inadequately or inappropriately prepared.*

The second factor that can contribute to ineffective teaching behaviors is the *conditioning processes that cause bad habits to become established and maintained.* New teachers, often formally unprepared, may develop bad habits due to the absence of role models or guidelines for effective teaching behaviors. Frequently, habits so developed are retained throughout a teaching career. Mentors or master teachers can be very important to new teachers in developing good teaching habits. While some schools now offer graduate students a teaching practicum, most do not. Departments or schools should provide some mechanism to help new teachers approach their teaching responsibilities.

For teachers who have taught for many years, early bad habits may have received years of reinforcement, making it even harder for them to change. It is difficult for teachers to recognize bad habits if there is *no mechanism for giving feedback to alert teachers to inappropriate behaviors.*

CONDUCTING A SELF-ANALYSIS

Whether using a formal or informal system of self-analysis, teachers should begin by assessing the following three areas: student characteristics, teacher characteristics, and developmental factors. Elements from each of these areas affect teachers' behaviors and attitudes, and therefore affect their participation in the teaching-learning process.

Student Characteristics

Before teachers can determine how they respond to different student characteristics, they need to be aware of the general ways in which specific student characteristics affect teachers. There is some data available, based largely on studies of precollege teaching-learning environments, which indicate that social-class differences, race, and student achievement all have an impact on teachers' behaviors and their attitudes toward students. Much research is needed in the area of teacher behavioral responses to these student characteristics, particularly in regard to postsecondary or adult students. The data that have been compiled, while not directly related to health science education, can be used as a general guideline for teachers' self-analysis.

Students' socioeconomic status can help predict teachers' perceptions of students and the way teachers treat students in the classroom. It has been shown that teachers view students from middle- and upper-income families more positively than they do students from lower-income families, and that they are more likely to praise and reward higher-status students, while giving more criticism and fewer rewards to lower-class students (8). Teachers become more concerned about instructing higher-status students, but at the same time feel responsible for controlling and disciplining lower-status students (6).

Race is another student characteristic that can have an effect on teacher behaviors and attitudes. Some teachers have more negative attitudes toward black students than they do toward white students (5). Inattention in a white student may be interpreted as an indication of the teacher's need to arouse student interest; the same behavior observed in a black student might be written off as boredom due to the student's "limited" attention span. Teachers are likely to have a subconscious negative bias toward minority students and treat them inappropriately in the classroom. Such responses are usually unconscious; in fact, many teachers indignantly deny the possibility of their treating students unequally.

Because teachers generally set high performance standards for themselves, they often expect students to strive to meet similarly high standards. Thus, it frequently happens that high-achieving students are viewed more positively and evaluated more positively than are low-achieving students (4). These kinds of reactions can serve implicitly to categorize students, often unfairly or inaccurately, so that, regardless of later work, a student who does poorly on a first examination may be consistently viewed as a low-ability student.

All teachers form opinions of their students. Some of these opinions are based on accurate perceptions, others on inaccurate or distorted perceptions. Teachers' opinions can also be based on their reactions to specific student characteristics. These opinions and perceptions contribute to the expectations teachers have for their classes and for specific students, and to teachers' subsequent behavior in the teaching-learning process. Because of the influence of their opinions and attitudes, it is crucial for teachers to honestly assess how they react to various student characteristics.

Teacher Characteristics

Teachers' self-analyses should also include an examination of their own characteristics as teachers. Several clusters of positive and negative, facilitating and inhibiting teacher characteristics have been identified. A synthesis of research results indicates, for example, that characteristics consistently associated with superior teachers or teaching include stimulation of interest, clarity of thought and expression, knowledge of subject matter, preparation for and organization of a course, and enthusiasm for subject matter and for teaching. Further, students consistently prefer teachers who demonstrate concern and respect for students, are available for advice and consultation without fostering dependent relationships, and are open to the opinions of others (3).

Teachers who facilitate students learning and creativity also have been described as accepting different or orthodox views; conducting classes in an informal yet well-prepared manner; emphasizing the understanding of principles; using student examinations as aids to learning and as evaluation tools; and as rewarding student initiative, originality, and creativity. Teachers who inhibit student learning and creativity, on the other hand, require students to memorize materials; de-emphasize independent study; rely on cynicism and sarcasm to handle students; spend little time with students outside of class; and show little toleration for disagreement with their views (2).

The inclusion of these teacher characteristics is intended to be illustrative only, not prescriptive, providing teachers with examples of behaviors they can use in their own self-analysis. Because interpretation of the presence or absence of these and similar characteristics is highly individualistic (e.g., what might be imaginative behavior for one teacher might be routine behavior for another), the assistance of colleagues in validating a teacher's self-analysis is essential. Thus, the teacher, in assessing personal teaching characteristics, should first complete a general self-assessment and then compare this assessment with one conducted by a trusted and respected colleague. Parallel student input in the form of formal or informal course evaluation is also very helpful.

Developmental Factors

A third area teachers should consider in conducting a self-assessment is that of personal developmental factors. At any point in time, teaching behaviors are a reflection of the teacher's personal development. For example, a teacher who is thirty years old may deal with issues of intimacy or authority differently than a teacher who is fifty years old; in developmental terms, their approaches to adult tasks are different.

Adult life is currently being studied carefully and several frameworks outlining various predictable adult stages have emerged (7). Such a framework—i.e., one that describes growth over the adult life span—can be helpful to the teacher. It can make the teacher aware, for example, that, during certain life stages, more interest and energy is likely to be available to devote to the role of teacher than during other times. The teacher equipped with such knowledge can plan to invest energy in reassessing and developing teacher skills at optimal times. Thus, while self-evaluation is a lifelong activity, certain times in one's life are better than others for focusing on self-improvement activities. These times should be identified, anticipated, and planned for by the individual teacher.

Teachers should never stop growing and changing. Each new teaching situation presents the opportunity to develop new insights into the process of teaching and the teacher as a person. Increased self-awareness can help the teacher develop a relationship with a student, participate in the student's growth and learning by both giving and receiving, and then terminate the relationship to begin another.

Self-awareness also allows teachers to develop trust rapidly with students. The more teachers understand their areas of limitations with students, the more easily teachers can manage students' testing behaviors. When students engage in testing by pointing out an error or an area of weakness, the self-aware teacher does not feel immediately defensive, having already been cognizant of the weakness and accepted it. It is the ability to be fully honest with students that allows teachers to develop the student-teacher relationship to its fullest.

A PERSONAL PLAN FOR DEVELOPMENT

Once the teacher has received feedback on student and teacher characteristics and has become familiar with the developmental factors of adulthood, a personal plan for development should be outlined. The personal plan reflects the present professional and personal status of the individual teacher. One teacher may feel the need to focus on skill development, for example, while another may decide to concentrate on personal awareness and insight.

Life management can facilitate implementation of the personal plan. As a health care professional enters the field of teaching, all of the stressors present in the field continue to be experienced, in addition to new stressors related to the role of teaching. As the professional continues in the field of teaching, job-related responsibilities usually increase further. Thus it can be anticipated that stress levels will increase simultaneously.

As a part of life management, teachers should address themselves to how they currently cope with stress and consider alternative ways of coping, on the assumption that stress is likely to increase. Certainly, if the teacher currently copes with stress by overeating, drinking, or smoking, now is a good time to look for alternative ways. In general, all teachers should strive to develop effective coping patterns.

Whenever possible the teacher should try to remove the source or manage the source of stress in life. A summer off, for example, could be exactly what the teacher needs to better cope during the remaining months. Often the stressors that teachers experience cannot be removed or reduced, however, so that additional measures to cope with them more adequately are desirable. Additional measures can be anything from a serious hobby or avocation to meditation, yoga, or routine exercise. The particular combination of measures used is not important. What is important is the teacher's ability to manage increasing stress more effectively, so there is energy left to devote to growth and development and the enjoyment of the teaching process.

The management of stress in a teacher's life should be considered in the general context of the teacher's health. Just as one's developmental tasks affect all areas of one's behavior, so too do physical and mental health. It is not just how one copes, but also how one feels physically. A teacher needs to accept that one can control to a large degree the level of well-being that is maintained. Routine health care and a concern for the quality of daily life can contribute greatly to how much energy a teacher has to offer a student and how much energy can be put into personal growth and development.

Teachers who are willing to put energy into managing their lives, so there is energy to continue to grow as a teacher, should anticipate a variety of reactions from peers, some of them negative. Some peers may feel threatened, simply because the changing and growing colleague makes them feel "inadequate" as teachers. The element of threat can be reduced substantially if the teacher who is able to grow and change makes it very clear to peers that what happens to work for one teacher is not necessarily appropriate for everyone else. It is sometimes helpful for the changing teacher to share mistakes, to keep peers informed of new teaching approaches, and to encourage positive signs of growth in them. In some situations, the resistance to change may be so great that the teacher will need to look outside the immediate environment for support and people with whom to share this new growth. Affiliation and support might be found in other areas of the school, in a special-interest group, or in a professional organization. A support system is necessary to implementing a personal development plan; a priority of the teacher should therefore be to locate and develop a support system of some kind.

When considering the teacher-self relationship, it is necessary for the teacher to assess several areas and to use personal insight and the insight of peers and students to formulate a plan for personal growth and development. The personal plan that is formulated and implemented within the context of the teacher's present life experience can contribute greatly to the teacher's ability to experience fully the demands and rewards of the teaching-learning process.

REFERENCES

1. BROPHY, JERE E. and THOMAS L. GOOD. *Teacher-Student Relationships: Causes and Consequences*. New York: Holt, Rinehart and Winston, 1974.

2. CHAMBERS, JACK A. "College Teachers: Their Effect on Creativity of Students." *Journal of Educational Psychology* 65 (1973): 326–334.

3. FELDMAN, KENNETH A. "The Superior College Teacher from the Students' View." *Research in Higher Education* 5 (1976): 243–288.

4. HOYT, DONALD P., and RONALD K. SEPANGLER. "Faculty Research Involvement and Instructional Outcomes." *Research in Higher Education* 4 (1976): 113–122.

5. LEACOCK, E. *Teaching and Learning in City Schools*. New York: Basic Books, 1969.

6. RIST, R. "Student Social-Class and Teacher Expectations: The Self-Fulfilling Prophecy in Ghetto Education." *Harvard Educational Review* 40 (1970): 411–451.

7. SHEEHY, GAIL. *Passages: Predictable Crises of the Adult Years*. New York: Bantam Books, 1976.

8. YEE, ARNOLD. "Interpersonal Attitudes of Teachers and Advantaged and Disadvantaged Pupils." *Journal of Human Resources* 3 (1968): 327–345.

UNIT 5
BIBLIOGRAPHY

BALDRIDGE, J. VICTOR, ed. *Academic Governance.* Berkeley: McCutchan, 1971.

A collection of research-based articles on institutional politics and decision making in higher education. While not directly related to health science education, the book provides a good diversity in points of view about various organizational processes in higher education. Essays in Part 2, "Administrative Processes," and those in Part 3, "The Faculty and the Governance Process," should be useful to anyone associated with a higher-education institution.

BROPHY, JERE E., and THOMAS L. GOOD. *Teacher-Student Relationships: Causes and Consequences.* New York: Holt, Rinehart and Winston, 1974.

In general, a good book on the research of student-teacher relationships in such areas as individual differences in teacher-student interaction patterns, the influences of the sex of the teacher and student on classroom behavior, individual differences and their implications for teachers and students. The chapter on teacher expectations is highly informative. The book also has a fine reference section.

KNIGHT, JAMES A. *Medical Student: Doctor in the Making.* New York: Appleton-Century-Crofts, 1973.

A psychiatrist-medical educator's descriptive analysis of the effects of the medical education process on students. Fast reading, informative; conveys sense of empathy for students, even for those who have not experienced the process.

LIKERT, RENSIS, and JANE GIBSON LIKERT. *New Ways of Managing Conflict.* New York: McGraw-Hill, 1976.

A systematic discussion of the causes, management, and resolution of conflict in organizations. Although directed principally at administrators or those in leadership positions, its management skills should be useful for anyone functioning in a formal organization.

ROGERS, CARL. *Freedom to Learn*. Columbus, Ohio: Merrill, 1969.

Establishes a person-oriented approach to the teaching-learning process. In the context of this approach, provides insight into the potential relationships teachers can develop with students.

SHEEHY, GAIL. *Passages: Predictable Crises of the Adult Years*. New York: Bantam Books, 1976.

Interesting book that examines adult life developmental passages with the objective of developing a framework for predicting these passages. Descriptive vignettes are very good.

TROLL, LILLIAN E. *Early and Middle Adulthood*. Monterey, Ca.: Brooks/Cole, 1975.

Excellent overview on the physical, intellectual, and personality development of the early and middle adult years. The book also presents content on the adult in terms of family development and in terms of the job world. Combines theory and empirical findings. Good resource for teachers of adult students.

WICKS, ROBERT J. *Counseling Strategies and Intervention Techniques for the Human Services*. Philadelphia: Lippincott, 1977.

Very basic book, but a good and quick review of interviewing and counseling strategies. Helpful to teachers counseling depressed or anxious students.

INDEX

Adjunct program
  form of learning package, 92
  form of programmed instruction, 75–76
Anxiety in groups, 139–140
Assessing group skills, 134
Assessment of student characteristics, 17,
    19, 43–51
  aid to planning instructional media, 59
  use in selecting learning activities, 96
Assessment of student learning
  formative, 171–173
    diagnostic test, 172
    prerequisite test, 171–172
    pretest, 172
    self-assessment test, 172–173
  summative, 173
    learning objectives related to, 173
  techniques, 173–184
    essay examinations, 180–182
    multiple-choice examinations,
      174–178
    oral examinations, 180, 182
    performance observation, 183–184
    projects, 182–183
    simulation exercises, 178–180
Associationist learning theory. *See*
    Teaching-learning process

Audiotapes, 71–73
  budget considerations, 72
  production, 72–73
  purpose, 71–72
  vignettes in, 72

Clinical survey, 114–115
Clinical teaching, 21, 113–121
  administrative planning, 117–118
  clinical schedules, 116–117
  definition, 21
  evaluation in, 120–121
  orientation to, 118
  planning for, 114
  pre- and postconferences, 117
  selecting, 115
  use of practice laboratory, 119–120
Cognitive learning theory. *See* Teaching-
    learning process
Cognitive preference style, 47–49
Cognitive style, 49–50
Contingency contracting, 127–129
  characteristics, 128
  guidelines for using, 127–128
  progress checks, 129
  rewards, types of, 129
Criterion-referenced measurement, 41, 170

Development
  definition, 18
  stage in teaching-learning process, 18-19
Developmental competence objectives,
    30-32. *See also* Learning objectives
Diagnosis phase of evaluation
    process. *See* Evaluation process

Essay examinations, 180-182
  extended-response question, 180-181
  restricted-response question, 180-181
Evaluation
  definition, 149
  phase in teaching-learning process,
    22-23
  types of, 150
    formative, 150
    summative, 150-151
Evaluation information, sources of,
    table, 159
Evaluation of material resources, 187-195
  colleague opinion, 194
  cost and cost benefit, 192-194
  experimental studies, 191
  practitioner opinion, 194-195
  student achievement information,
    187-188
  student opinion, 188-189
  teacher observation, 191-192
Evaluation plan, guidelines for
    developing, 17, 41-42
Evaluation process, phases of,
    22, 153-166
  examination, 22, 153, 154-163
  diagnosis, 22, 153, 163-165
  prescription, 22, 153, 165-166
  summary, table of, 154
Evaluation of student learning. *See*
    Assessment of student learning
Evaluation of teacher performance,
    197-200
  colleague observation, 199
  practitioner observation, 199-200
  student opinion, 197-198
  teacher self-analysis, 198-199
  microteaching, 198

Evaluation of teaching-learning activities
    195-197
  colleague observation, 197
  practitioner observation, 197
  student information, 196
  teacher observation, 196-197
Examination phase of evaluation process.
    See Evaluation process
Experiential learning. *See* Learning

Formative assessment of student learning.
    See Assessment of student learning
Formative evaluation. *See* Evaluation

Goals, instructional, 15, 28-29
  definition, 15
  examples, 15, 29
Grades, 170
Group experiences
  advantages of, 133
  disadvantages of, 133
  importance for developmental
      competence objectives, 134
Group life
  phases, 5-7, 134-137
    initiation, 5-6, 134-136
    termination, 6-7, 137
    working, 6, 136-137
Group skills
  assessing, 134
  developing, 137-141
Groups
  anger in, 140
  anxiety in, 139-140
  heterogeneous, 35
  homogeneous, 36
  honesty in, 140
  leading, 21
  orientation to purpose, 134-136
  phases of, table, 135
  silence in, 140
  testing behaviors, 5, 136, 139-141

Initiation phase of group life. *See*
    Group life
Instruction, personalized. *See*
    Personalized instruction

Instruction, programmed. *See*
  Programmed instruction
Instructional goals. *See* Goals,
  instructional
Instructional media, 57–77
  as "active carrier" of learning
    conditions, 60–61
  evaluating, 59–60
  guidelines for developing, 62–64
  as "passive carrier" of learning
    conditions, 60–61
  preview process for commercial media,
    63–64
  production budget, 66–67, 68, 72, 73,
    75
  selecting appropriate form, 60–62
  steps in planning for, 58–60
Instructional methods and materials
  selecting, 17, 39–41
  preparing, 19
Instructional time
  allocating, 38–39
    according to student characteristics,
      38–39
    according to type of learning
      objective, 38
  definition, 16
Interpersonal simulation games, 82
Item difficulty, 176, 204
Item discrimination, 176, 204

Laboratory teaching
  purpose, 21
  structured laboratory experience
    121–122
  unstructured laboratory experience,
    121–123
Large-system simulation games, 82
Learning
  experiential, 80
  theories. *See* Teaching-learning process
Learning objectives, 15, 29–32
  definition, 15
  developmental competence objectives
    assessed through projects, 182
    assessment methods for, 170

and criteria for evaluating student
  performance, 160, 176, 180, 182
function of, 30–32
importance of group experiences for,
  134
included in learning packages, 95
use in planning instructional media,
  59
example, 15
and formative assessment of student
  learning, 171–173
minimal competence objectives
  assessment methods for, 170
  and criteria for evaluating student
    performance, 160, 176, 180
  function of, 29–30
  included in learning packages, 95
  use in planning instructional media,
    58–59
and summative assessment of student
  learning, 173
Learning packages
  components, 94–98
    assessment devices, 95–96
    learning activities, 96–97
    learning objectives, 95
    prerequisites, 95
    resource materials, 98
  definition, 91–92
  developing a course composed of,
    99–100
  use in personalizing instruction, 126–127
Learning style, 46–47
Lecture, 20, 106–110
  effect of teacher's personal attributes
    on, 109
  purpose, 20, 107
  "spurt-sag-spurt" phenomenon, 108
  structure, 108
  students as active participants in, 109
Life management, 236–237

Management
  definition, 20
  stage in teaching-learning process, 19–22
Material resources, evaluation of. *See*
  Evaluation of material resources

Media, instructional. *See* Instructional media
Microteaching, 198. *See also* Evaluation of teacher performance; Self-analysis
Minimal competence objectives, 29–30. *See also* Learning objectives
Modules, use in managing laboratory experiences, 122–123
Motivation, process theory of, 217–218
Multiple-choice examinations, 174–178
  inappropriate uses of, 174
  performance standards for, 175–178
  reasons for widespread use of, 174
  table of specifications for, 175–176

Norm-referenced measurement, 41, 170
Nonsimulation games, 81

Objectives, learning. *See* Learning objectives
Objectivity, in interpreting evaluation results, 164
Oral examinations, 180, 182

Pacing, in slide-tapes, 71
Patient management problem. *See* Simulation exercise
Performance observation, 183–184
  method of conducting, 184
Performance standards
  designating item difficulty levels, 176–178
  for extended-response essay questions, 180
  for multiple-choice examinations, 175–178
  for observing student performance, 183
  for projects, 182
  for restricted-response essay questions, 180
  for simulation exercises, 179–180
  table of specifications, 175–176
Personalized instruction, 125–131
  contingency contracting, 127–129
  continuum for managing, 125

  definition, 125
  learning packages and, 126–127
  tutoring, 129–131
Planning
  definition, 13
  stage in teaching-learning process, 14–17
Planning exercises, 81
Prescription phase of evaluation process. *See* Evaluation process
Pretest
  assessment device in learning package, 95
  as formative assessment, 172
Programmed instruction, 74–76
  budget considerations, 75
  evaluating existing materials, 75
  production, 75–76
  purposes, 74
Projects, 182–183

Questionnaires, guidelines for constructing, 189–191

Reliability, 152, 205–209
  procedures for determining, 205–209
    coefficient alpha, 207–208
    coefficient of reproducibility, 208–209
    for developmental competence examinations, 206
    for minimal competence examinations, 205–206
    for subjective assessments, 207

Schedule of course meetings, arranging, 18
Script, 69–70
  flowchart for slide-tape production, illus., 70
Self-analysis, 138–139, 232–236
  areas of assessment, 233–236
    developmental factors, 235–236
    student characteristics, 233–234
    teacher characteristics, 234–235
Self-assessment
  in learning package, 96
  as formative assessment, 172–173

Seminar/discussions, 20. *See also* Small
    group discussion
Simulation exercises, 178–180
  advantages of, 178
  developing, 179
  limitations of, 179
  performance standard for, 179–180
Simulation games, 78–89
  applications, a comparison, table,
    83–84
  categories, 81–84
    interpersonal simulation games, 82
    large-system simulation games, 82
    nonsimulation games, 81
    planning exercises, 81
  designing and constructing, 86–87
  evaluating externally produced, 85–86
  functions of, 79–80
  timing of, 88
Slide-tapes, 68–71
  budget considerations, 68
  production, 69–71
  purpose, 68
  visuals, 70
Small-group discussion, 110–113
  composition of group, 112
  and developmental competence
    objectives, 110
  leadership of group, 113
  plan for, 111–112
"Spurt-sag-spurt" phenomenon. *See*
    Lecture
Storyboard, 67–68
Students
  dishonest, 220–221
  immature, 218–219
  mature, 219–220
  unmotivated, 216–218
  with emotional problems, 221–222
Study skills, 45–46
Subject content, 15, 32–34
  definition, 16
  selecting, 32–34
  sequencing, 16, 34–35
Summative assessment of student learning.
    See Assessment of student learning
Summative evaluation. *See* Evaluation

Syllabus
  definition, 91
  elements of, 92–93

Table of specifications, 171, 175–176
  example, 175
Teacher-Peer relationships, 223–231
  between teacher and administrative
    head, 227–228
  between teachers and assistants,
    228–229
  stages of, 223–226
  within institutional framework, 230–231
Teacher performance, evaluation of.
    See Evaluation of teacher
    performance
Teaching-learning activities, evaluation of.
    See Evaluation of teaching-
    learning activities
Teaching-learning process
  associationist approach, 9–11
    minimal competence objectives
      and, 30
    stimulus-response, 12
    teacher-centered classroom, 10
  cognitive approach, 11–13
    developmental competence objectives
      and, 31
    problem solving, 12
    student-centered classroom, 11
  stages of, 13
Team teaching, 226–227
Termination phase of group life, 6–7, 137
"Testing" behaviors, 5
  in teacher-peer relationships, 224
  means to establish trust in groups,
    136–141
Tests, achievement. *See* Assessment of
    student learning
Transparencies for overhead projection,
    73–74
  budget considerations, 73
  production, 73–74
  purpose, 73
Trust
  between teacher and students, 5, 17,
    39, 126–127

established during initiation phase of
group life, 134–136
in teacher-peer relationships, 224
Tutoring, 120–131
procedures in developing tutoring
schedule, 130

Unsafe behavior, 120

Validity, 151–152, 201–205
construct validity, 202

content validity, 202–203
criterion-related validity, 202
procedures for determining, 203–205
item analysis statistics, 204–205
validity index, 203
Value judgments, 165–166
Videotape, 64–68
budget considerations, 66–67
production, 67–68
purpose, 65

Working phase of group life, 6, 136–137